T0285666

The Voice of the Body

Books by Alexander Lowen, M.D.

The Language of the Body
  originally published as *Physical Dynamics of Character Structure*

Love and Orgasm: A Revolutionary Guide to Sexual Fulfillment

The Betrayal of the Body

Pleasure: A Creative Approach to Life

*Bioenergetics: The Revolutionary Therapy That Uses the Language of the Body
  to Heal the Problems of the Mind*

Depression and the Body: The Biological Basis of Faith and Reality

The Way to Vibrant Health: A Manual of Bioenergetic Exercises,
  co-author Leslie Lowen

Fear of Life

Narcissism: Denial of the True Self

Love, Sex, and Your Heart

The Spirituality of the Body: Bioenergetics for Grace and Harmony

Joy: The Surrender to the Body and to Life

Honoring the Body: The Autobiography of Alexander Lowen, M.D.

The Voice of the Body: Selected Public Lectures 1962-1982

LowenCorp Publishing LLC
Vermont, USA

The Voice of the Body

Selected Public Lectures 1962-1982
Alexander Lowen, M.D.

The Alexander Lowen Foundation
www.lowenfoundation.org

The Voice of The Body

Published by The Alexander Lowen Foundation
Shelburne, VT 05482
USA
www.lowenfoundation.org

Copyright © 2005 by Alexander Lowen, M.D.

All rights reserved. No part of this book may be reproduced or transmitted in
any form or by any means, electronic or mechanical, including photo-copying,
recording or by any information storage and retrieval system, without
permission in writing from the Publisher.

Except in the United States of America, this book is sold subject to the
condition that it shall not, by way of trade or otherwise, be lent, re-sold, hired
out, or otherwise circulated without the publisher's prior consent in any form of
binding or cover other than that in which it is published and without a
similar condition including this condition being imposed
on the subsequent publisher.

Library of Congress Control Number 2004104277
ISBN 978-1-938485-04-6 (paperback)
ISBN 978-1-938485-05-3 (ebook)

First Edition by The Alexander Lowen Foundation, 2012
New printing, February 2022
Printed in the United States of America

Contents

Preface

Alexander Lowen, M.D. invented Bioenergetic Analysis, a pioneering approach to psychotherapy that combines physical with psychological interventions. In this psychotherapy, information from patients' bodies, such as muscle tension patterns, is used diagnostically, while physical interventions are used to facilitate changes in patients' bodies and to increase their psychological awareness of conflicts that manifest in their bodies. Psychological information likewise guides the diagnostic process, while psychological interventions are used to facilitate physical changes in patients' bodies and to solidify psychological changes made through physical interventions. In this regard, Bioenergetic Analysis is truly a humanistic mind-body therapy that equally honors the physical and mental aspects of the whole person.

Lowen studied with the famed psychoanalyst, Wilhelm Reich, who in turn had studied directly with Sigmund Freud. Freud was known for frequently stating that the ego is fundamentally a body ego but the psychoanalysis he developed paid little attention to the body. Reich, however, took Freud's insight about the body's role in psychopathology further and developed a variety of psychotherapeutic approaches that relied on working with patients' bodies. Similarly, Lowen extended this tradition through his development of Bioenergetic Analysis.

This volume contains a collection of previously unpublished writings and lectures by Lowen that have informally been known for many years by bioenergetic practitioners as the "Lowen Monographs." These have been in private circulation through various pamphlets available through the International Institute for Bioenergetics and contain some of Lowen's most important and insightful ideas. By bringing these together in one volume, an important gap in the literature on bioenergetics is rectified. In order for these to be made accessible to the general reader, they are ordered with more specialized topics presented last rather than chronologically.

In "Stress and Illness: A Bioenergetic View," Lowen outlines a theory of illness applicable to what has conventionally been seen as either physical or mental diseases, demonstrating the inadequacies of a mind-body dualism that categorizes in such mutually exclusive ways. Instead, he presents these as psychosomatic, combining elements of mind and body in all instances. Lowen discusses psychological variables germane to both treatment and prevention of many so-called physical illnesses, reinforcing the importance of holding a unified view of mind and body.

In "The Rhythm of Life," Lowen explores pleasure in relationship to the body. Whereas illness and disease are often seen as substantial, Lowed notes how pleasure is frequently seen as insubstantial and elusive. He outlines an embodied theory of pleasure based on body rhythms that goes much further than defining it as merely the absence of pain. His discussion includes a theory of emotions focusing on the deleterious consequences of their repression, ending in consideration of the energy field that surrounds and interconnects us all.

In "Breathing, Movement, and Feeling," Lowen takes this notion of rhythm further through focusing on breathing and movement, fundamental rhythmic processes essential to life that determine feeling. He presents a number of therapeutic exercises to deepen feelings and discusses the importance of expression of repressed negative feelings as the starting place of therapy.

This theme is expanded in "Self-Expression: New Developments in Bioenergetic Therapy." Lowen emphasizes how self-expression is fundamentally movement. He also focuses on the importance of the eyes in both self-expression and making contact with others. This discussion includes a psychological theory of eye disorders, along with Lowen's view of emotional health as based on the degree of expression that can be sustained through eye contact with others.

In "Thinking and Feeling: The Bioenergetic Analysis of Thought," Lowen explores the role of thought in relationship to emotions, including its adaptive function and its capacity for being distorted as a defense mechanism. He considers the role of thought as especially important in self-assertion through maintaining a critical rationality. Likewise, the relationship between thought and both truth and beauty are explored.

In "Sex and Personality," Lowen presents a view of sexuality related to human evolution that ultimately is essential in overcoming the sense of isolation and loneliness incumbent with individuation. He develops this into a comparison of the dynamics of homosexuality, as contrasted with heterosexuality, as well as a theory of orgastic experience, including its differential expression in males and females.

In "The Will to Live and the Wish to Die" Lowen theorizes how both concepts can pose resistances prohibiting fulfillment in life. Obviously an orientation toward seeking death, as expressed in suicidal ideation, is such a barrier; however, Lowen demonstrates how the will to live can also be a similar obstacle in terms of denial of our human predicament. Invoking the importance of accessing aggression in service of our fulfillment, Lowen proposes a way to reconcile this predicament.

Lowen develops this theme of life and death struggles further in "Horror: The Face of Unreality and Self-Expression vs. Survival." Defined as a sense of shock, horror is portrayed as culturally endemic and deadening of feelings. Lowen explores how self-expression can be seen as the escape from being deadened by horror.

In "Aggression and Violence in the Individual," Lowen explores distinctions between aggression and both violence and cruelty. These are discussed in terms of how people can be literally "hung-up," namely cut-off from their lower body, such as their bowels and genitals, and the role of the lower body in aggression and violence.

Finally, in "Psychopathic Behavior and the Psychopathic Personality," Lowen theorizes about the role of power and control in relationship to empty, frustrating, and self-defeating lifestyles. The psychopath is viewed as emphasizing manipulation and focusing on the goal of self-elevation while ignoring the harmful means by which this is achieved.

In conclusion, this collection of writings by Lowen addresses bioenergetic approaches to many areas not covered in his other published books and often provides for areas that are covered elsewhere a greater depth and breadth of coverage. Anyone seriously interested in bioenergetic analysis, or the wider field of mind-body therapies (sometimes known as "somatics") could benefit greatly from Lowen's brilliant insights in these monographs. It is especially timely to present this collection now, closely following the publication of Lowen's long-awaited autobiography, *Honoring the Body*. Finally, I want to thank Alexander Lowen for his making these monographs available for publication and Robert Glazer, Ph.D., President of the Florida Society for Bioenergetic Analysis, for inviting me to edit these works.

Harris Friedman, Ph.D., Editor
Professor Emeritus, Saybrook Graduate School
Professor (Courtesy), University of Florida
Certified Bioenergetic Therapist and Florida Licensed Psychologist

Lectures

Lectures given at the Hotel Biltmore, New York City
1965—Breathing, Movement, and Feeling: The Basis of Bioenergetic Analysis

Lectures given at the Community Church, New York City
1962—Sex and Personality: A Study in Orgastic Potency
1966—The Rhythm of Life: A Discussion of the Relation between Pleasure and Rhythmic Activities of the Body
1967—Thinking and Feeling: The Bioenergetic Analysis of Thought
1968—Self-Expression: New Developments in Bioenergetic Therapy
1969—Aggression and Violence in the Individual
1972-1973—Horror: The Face of Unreality /
        Self-Expression vs. Survival
1975—Psychopathic Behavior and the Psychopathic Personality

Other Lectures
1980—Stress and Illness: A Bioenergetic View
1982—The Will To Live and the Wish to Die

1

Stress and Illness:
A Bioenergetic View

THE NATURE OF ILLNESS

This lecture stems from my interest in psychosomatic illnesses such as arthritis, ulcerative colitis, coronary heart disease, lupus erythematosus, psoriasis, migraine, etc. Over the years I have treated a number of patients with these diseases with some success. I have also had many failures which have forced me to think about the nature of these illnesses. One observation has impressed me. Some persons are more prone to somatic illness while others are more prone to mental illness. It appears that there is some degree of exclusivity between these two kinds of response to trauma or stress. On the other hand I have long maintained that all illness is psychosomatic since psyche and soma are only two different faces of an organism's functioning. This seeming contradiction can be explained by Wilhelm Reich's statement that psyche and soma are both antithetical and functionally identical. Their function is identical on the energetic level on which level we can best comprehend the body's reaction to stress.

That all illness may be seen as a reaction to stress is not a new concept. The role of stress in the etiology of certain chronic illnesses was beautifully shown by Hans Seyle, a pioneer in this field. However, to justify the statement that all illness is related to stress, we have to extend the concept of stress to include such situations as invasion by parasites or pathological micro-organisms and even accidents. For example, if a person sprains his ankle, he becomes ill (as opposed to being well) because the resulting swelling and pain prevents him from walking normally. The stress in this case is the sprained ligament to which the body reacts with swelling and pain. The accident is the stressor agent which produces the stress, which, in turn, causes the reaction we call illness. If the sprain is mild and does not result in swelling and pain, the person would not be considered ill.

Pathogenic bacteria are also stressor agents when they invade the body putting it under stress. In this case, too, the stress may be mild causing little reaction from the body. Or it may be fairly severe if the bacteria are virulent and result in illness marked by fever, inflammation and weakness. If the body can cope with the stress caused by a stressor agent without markedly disturbing its normal functioning, there is no illness. Illness in this sense is equivalent to dis-ease and represents a breakdown of the body's normal functioning. It always denotes an inability of the body to cope with a stress.

Here is another example. Recently I suffered from an attack of poison ivy. Of course, I wasn't attacked. I simply touched the roots of the poison ivy plant which exudes an oily substance that is slightly toxic to the skin. Both of my forearms reacted after several days with a rash, swelling and intense itching. Localized areas of inflammation appeared on other parts of my body which also itched fiercely. I finally had a shot of cortisone which quickly reduced the swelling but the itching diminished only slowly. The illness in this case was the body's reaction to the stress caused by the poison ivy exudate which was the stressor agent. The rash, inflammation and itching represented the body's attempt which was the stressor agent. The rash, inflammation and itching represented the body's attempt to overcome or remove the stressor agent and to repair the damage it caused. However, there have been other occasions when I was exposed to poison ivy and did not react with illness. In those cases my body coped with the stress without upsetting my well-being.

Note that there is always some delay between the exposure to a stressor agent and the reaction to the stress it causes. That needs to be explained. Have you noticed that when you are cut by a very sharp instrument, there is no pain at the moment of the trauma? The pain sets in seconds later. The explanation is that the injury produces a momentary state of shock in the organism. The pain supervenes only when the shock wears off and the body reacts with an exudation of fluid to heal the wound. The exudate slowly thickens and hardens to cover the break in the surface of the organism. Later it becomes a scab. In this situation, the pain is due to the pressure created when the flow of blood, fluid and energy meets the resistance of the break. Pain must be viewed as a positive life expression. There is no pain in death nor in dying. It is the struggle against dying that causes pain. To understand pain as the result of a vital force against a block or resistance, consider the pain of childbirth when the baby's head is pressing against an undilated cervix. A similar condition develops when a large and hard fecal mass is being pushed through a tight anal orifice. A block or contraction is not painful when no force or energy is directed against it. On the other hand, when there is no resistance to the force or energy, the result is a flow that is pleasurable. The best illustration of this concept is the phenomenon of frostbite. When a part of the body suffers frostbite, there is no pain. The pain supervenes when the part is being warmed. It is due to the pressure caused by the flow of blood into the frozen and contracted tissues. Thawing out a frost-bitten finger or hand must be done very gradually to avoid the extreme pain and the danger of damage to the cells from the pressure. The immediate reaction to every trauma is shock which may go so far as to result in a loss of consciousness. It is only as the shock wears off and the body reacts positively to the trauma that pain develops. The same thing is true of inflammation.

An illness must be viewed, therefore, as the body's attempt to restore its integrity following some trauma. I first heard this view expressed by my professor of pathology in medical school. I have since learned that it was the common view of nineteenth century medicine and stemmed from Claude Bernard's concept of disease as the outcome of the body's attempt at homeostasis in which the adaptive response to a noxious force is inadequate. I believe it is a basic medical concept. The word trauma can include any injury to the organism. It is equivalent to an overwhelming stress no matter what the nature of the stressor agent. If the body cannot arrive at coping with the stress, the illness will end in the death of the organism.

Stress does not necessarily result in illness. We are subject to many stresses in life which we can take in our stride. The organism is capable of handling the common stresses of its life situation without any disruption of its normal functioning. Every weight that one picks up produces a stress in the body yet we pick up heavy objects all the time without any problem. But sometimes the weight is too heavy or too awkward and we injure ourselves. In that case the stress was more than we could handle. It happened to me a short time ago.

I wanted to change the wheels on my car and so I applied the lug wrench to one of the bolts. Sensing that it was stuck I gave the wrench a strong upward jerk. The bolt held and the car almost came off the ground and I heard something in my back go c-r-u-n-c-h. I knew that I had damaged my back but I felt no pain and so continued to work. I loosened the bolts by kicking the wrench with my foot and so I was able to change all the wheels. When I finished, my back felt stiff but I was able to straighten up and move about without pain. I experienced some stiffness in my lower back for about a week but with the bioenergetic exercises it disappeared. About three weeks later, I felt very anxious in my pelvic floor with unpleasant, prickly sensations which were very uncomfortable. They left after a day and a half. Then several days later my hip began to hurt me.

For the next three months, I had pain in my right hip often shooting down my leg. It hurt whenever I moved my pelvis backward as in sex. The pain seemed to be localized deep in the right buttocks extending upward to the lumbosacral area. I had trouble turning over in bed. In the morning when I got up, I could hardly stand on my right leg. At times

I walked with a slight limp. The pain and distress was always worse in the morning but doing the bioenergetic exercises relieved the pain and I could move about fairly freely. I continued to attend the bioenergetic exercise classes but I had to go easy. When the pain became strong, I would stop. I also had my regular massages but less frequently since it was summertime. On one occasion I had my masseuse dig into the right buttocks but the result was disastrous. For two days afterward the pain was quite severe. I had thought the maneuver would relax the tight muscles but it didn't. However, the experience convinced me that the deep pelvic muscles were in a state of spasm and they would need considerable time to relax. Actually, my whole right side was involved for there was a noticeably increased state of tension in my right side extending from the kidney area to the foot.

I didn't go to a doctor because I don't believe they understand the nature of lower back pain. Since I was not incapacitated I was reluctant to put myself in their hands. I do not like to surrender the responsibility for my body to anyone else. As long as I could move about I trusted that my body would heal itself. Further, I am not terrified by pain for I recognize that it is part of the healing process. However, when the illness continued without major improvement, I did see two chiropractors. Given the sound I heard at the moment of the accident, I thought it likely that I had slightly displaced a vertebra. The first man did some tests which indicated to him that I may have herniated the disk between L4 and L5. He did some gentle maneuvers while I was on the chiropractic table, but I seemed to get most relief from the application of heat to the painful area in the buttocks. I felt somewhat better after the treatment but the pain returned the next day. I did not follow up the treatment with him despite his suggestion that I do so. His diagnosis was that I had a case of sciatica due to pressure on the sciatic nerve. I agreed with his diagnosis. And, since the sciatica continued, I saw another recommended chiropractor one month later. He confirmed the diagnosis but he located the lesion, slipped disk, between L5 and Sl. His maneuver was to push the right side of the pelvis backward which produced a slight clicking sound. I felt a little better after this treatment. He, too, counseled further treatment which I did not pursue.

I kept doing the exercises and having my massages and the sciatic pain lessened. In October, I saw Dr. McIntyre and he told me that he had heard from some orthopedic men that the pressure on the sciatic nerve which caused the pain in the leg was due to a spasm of the glutens medius muscle which compressed the nerve as it passed through the sciatic notch. That was where I always felt the most pain. He said that it was advised that one bend forward, straightening the knees to stretch the hamstring muscles. This is similar to the bioenergetic exercise I was doing. I had felt all along that I needed to pull the pelvis backward to release the spasm and this is what the bending forward exercise accomplishes. But it was in the act of sex that I felt something let go as I pulled the pelvis backward. This had been the position of most pain previously. From that moment on I have been completely free from any pain in my back, buttocks or leg. In fact I feel freer in that region than before because of the attention I was forced to give to it.

Thinking about the event that caused my sciatica I realized that it was not simply an accident. I knew better than to do what I did. I knew that my legs should be bent to take the pressure when lifting a weight or exerting an upward force. I could only conclude that my action was designed, unconsciously, to injure myself. Why? Well, despite all the work I had done with my body bioenergetically, I was somewhat out of touch with the tension in my lower back. The injury focused my attention on that area, as I mentioned above, and made me work more intensively with it. And it also made me more conscious of my tendency to force situations. I am predominantly right handed and right sided. The pain in my right leg forced me to put my weight on my left leg which helped to balance my body and my personality. Not all injuries turn out to have such positive benefits but then, most people are out of touch with their bodies and their personalities. Most people are terrified by pain and so avoid every painful situation. They do not appreciate that pain is a positive response of the body to stress.

When the body is *overpowered* by a stressor agent its first reaction is shock, which consists of the withdrawal of energy and blood from the surface of the body, the skin, mucous membranes and striated musculature. The shock can be localized, as in the case of a small cut, but most often it is a general reaction. This withdrawal of energy explains why hair can turn white after a shock. The hair becomes dark again when the energy returns to the hair follicles. This sequence of shock, (withdrawal of energy) and rebound, (return of energy) is characteristic, I believe, of the onset of all illness. It is seen most clearly in the common cold. My colds often start with a sore throat (upper respiratory inflammation). I treat it by going to bed and sweating it out. I take some aspirin, drink hot tea and cover myself well. As the sore throat subsides I develop a head cold which may run for a couple of days. And "run" is what my nose does before it dries up.

Two factors always operate to produce a cold in me. The first is tiredness. If I chill off when I am tired, I catch a cold. This does not happen when I am rested. Tiredness indicates that my resistance is low; it means that my energy is temporarily depleted. The second factor is stress. The stress could be due to a physical chill (exposure to cold), an emotional chill or an extra exertion like a speaking engagement. What about the role of the cold virus? I believe that the virus is present in the body at all times following our first exposure to it as infants or children. Normally, it is not active. One's resistance is high, we say.

It generally takes several days after exposure to the stressor agent for a cold to develop. What is going on in this time? Some might say that it is a period of incubation. I think I can offer a better explanation. The "cold" begins with a chill and ends in a heat. The chill is an actual lowering of the body temperature. The body may then respond with a fever to overcome the chilling. I try to raise my body temperature by external means. The chilling of the body results from the state of shock, the withdrawal of blood and energy from the surface of the body, including the mucous membranes of the upper respiratory tract. The cells of this mucous lining become contracted and frozen. In the body's rebound from the state of shock, blood and energy flow back into the mucous lining of the throat "exploding" the frozen cells. (The burning pain of a severe sore throat is like the burning pain of a frost-bitten finger when it is warmed too quickly.) They disintegrate and are replaced by new cells. The detritus has to be removed which creates the often purulent discharge. The death and disintegration of the frozen cells is somehow related to the proliferation of the virus.

Seen in the light of the above, a cold has two stages. During the presymptomatic days the tissues are in a state of freeze and the body in a state of shock. Then a thaw sets in, symptoms appear and the nose starts to run. It is similar to the spring thaw of a frozen stream. Freeze and thaw correspond to shock and rebound. Have you noticed that when a cold has run its course you feel renewed? In part this is due to the rest enforced by the cold, but the energetic rebound from the shock also plays a part. If one aborts the symptoms, one risks to remain in the tired state and be vulnerable to more serious illness.

The common cold offers much to the student of psychosomatic illness. For one thing, there seems to be an inverse relationship between catching cold and becoming depressed. I used to catch cold easily but I rarely got depressed. The common element in both the cold and the depressive reaction is a state of energy depletion (tiredness, exhaustion). But why one person catches a cold while another gets depressed in this condition is a question I will answer later. The other interesting aspect of the common cold is that it rarely affects schizophrenics. In fact, when one of these individuals develops a cold, it is a sign of improvement in his state of mental health.

The explanation for the schizophrenic's seeming resistance to the common cold is that he is in a perpetual state of shock. I have previously described his condition as "frozen." Thus, he doesn't react to the cold or a chill as other people do. This was clearly illustrated by a young woman who had walked through the snow-covered streets of New York to my office wearing a pair of canvas sneakers. They were soaked and her feet were blue from the cold. She didn't sense it because she was numb to her body and in her body. She was frozen. She ended in a mental hospital with a diagnosis of schizophrenia. Another person in her situation would have ended in a general hospital with a diagnosis of pneumonia. When a schizophrenic person begins to thaw out from his generalized freeze, that is, become more responsive, he develops the symptoms of a cold when be becomes tired and chilled.

THE NATURE OF STRESS

In the preceding section I spoke of stress in general terms. If we are to apply our bioenergetic understanding to the relation of stress to illness, the former term should be defined energetically. But first, let us look at its common usage which derives from mechanics. In physics, stress denotes the operation of a force which subjects a body or object to strain or deformation. Harold G. Wolfe, whose book *Stress and Disease* was published in 1953, defines stress as "the *interaction* between external environment and organism." The strain is the effect upon the organism. He then says, "The magnitude of the latter and the capacity of the organism to withstand the strain determine whether or not there will be re-establishment of homeostasis or a 'break,' with disruption and death."[1]

For Wolfe, the nature of the organism's reaction to stress was determined by its past experience. Thus, one person may react to overwhelming stress with arthritis while another may develop ulcerative colitis. A slightly different view was expressed by Hans Seyle, who was also studying the organism's reaction to stress. He believed that the organism's reaction to stress was non-specific; that is, the organism reacted the same to all stressor agents regardless of their nature. This reaction consisted of a hyperactivity of the adrenal cortex, a shrinkage of the thymus and lymph nodes and the development of gastric ulcers. He named this response the alarm reaction. Accordingly, he defined stress as a body state "manifested by a specific syndrome which consists of all the nonspecific induced changes in a biological system."[2] I do not see a basic disagreement between these two views. I believe that there is both a non-specific and a specific response to stress. One can focus upon either aspect.

Seyle's view of stress described above pictures it as a negative phenomenon. But since life does not and cannot exist without stress, such a view is too narrow. In 1974 in a book entitled *Stress Without Distress*[3] Seyle modified his position. He distinguished between stress and distress identifying the latter with pathology. Stress without distress, he stated, was not harmful to the organism and could even be used constructively. Most of us would agree with the distinction between stress and distress. We accept many stressful situations as challenging and exciting. Meeting the challenge often yields a deep satisfaction. For example, many people find that sailing a boat in rough weather, though stressful, is an exhilarating experience that promotes one's well-being. Other persons, however, may be frightened by this situation and find themselves exhausted by the experience. Obviously, if one can handle the stressful situation with some ease, the outcome is positive. If not, the situation becomes traumatic and the distress leads to dis-ease. In line with this distinction, Seyle modified his earlier definition of stress and redefined it as "the non-specific response of the body to any demand made upon it."[4]

This non-specific response can be none other than the expenditure of energy by the organism in response to demands made upon it. Natural forces in the environment such as gravity and the weather are constantly demanding an expenditure of energy by the organism. Even the simple maintenance of life functions requires the expenditure of energy. It takes energy to keep the heart pumping, the muscles contracting, the kidneys excreting, etc. As Albert Szent-Gyorgyi remarked, it takes energy to run the machine of life. In this sense we are under stress all the time. But the living body can cope with these stresses and others because it is producing energy all the time through its metabolic processes. In fact organisms, until they are old, produce an excess of energy for growth, for reproductive needs and to create a reserve. As long as a body has enough energy to meet the demands made upon it, it stays free from distress. A situation becomes distressing when it requires more energy than the body has available. By the same token any outside force that interferes with the body's ability to produce energy could throw it into distress. Thus, any serious interference with breathing creates an immediate sense of distress.

Seyle's great contribution to our understanding of stress is the formulation of the general adaptation syndrome which he abbreviated as the G.A.S. In a number of experiments he showed that when an organism is exposed to an overwhelming stress, it responds, as was noted above, with a hyperactivity of the adrenal cortex, a shrinkage of the thymus and lymph nodes, and the development of gastric ulcers. This initial response he called the alarm reaction. If the stress continues, the organism develops a resistance to the stress. The alarm reaction disappears. The organism has made a seemingly adequate adaptation to the stressful situation. Seyle called this second reaction the stage of resistance. However, if the situation continues to remain unchanged, the organism's resistance eventually collapses. It exhausts its reserve of what Seyle called its "adaptation energy" and dies. This third stage of the G.A.S. was named the stage of exhaustion. Seyle showed that every condition of stress (overwhelming stress), regardless of the nature of the stressor agent, produced the same sequence of events. For example, when a laboratory animal is exposed to excessive cold, it responds with an alarm reaction. Continued exposure results in an adaptation, the animal seems to tolerate the cold without ill effects. However, this tolerance is limited. In time the resistance diminishes and the animal succumbs.

The G.A.S. describes an energetic process. However, to reformulate that concept in energetic terms requires some clarification in the early sequence of events surrounding an overwhelming stress or trauma. Such a stress or trauma constitutes a threat to the integrity of the organism to which it reacts with shock. Now, shock is caused by the withdrawal of energy and blood from the periphery of the body or from the threatened or attacked area. Without the concept of shock it is difficult to understand the seemingly over-reaction of the body to rather innocuous stimuli like allergens or the discussion of emotional problems. The shock can be fatal if the trauma is severe enough. If not, the body rebounds from the shock and attempts to change or control the distressing situation. The physiological response to the shock is the alarm reaction. The body mobilizes its energy to meet the threat. Energy and blood flow back to the shocked or traumatized areas causing inflammation and pain. The development of fever is also an expression of energy mobilization.

If the distressing situation cannot be controlled or removed, the organism adapts to it by the continued use of reserve energy. The adaptation eliminates the experience of distress but the body remains under considerable stress; and while not in a state of disease (illness), it is not in a state of ease, either. Because one's reserve of energy is being used to maintain the adaptation, an additional shock could lead to illness. In any event, one's resistance is limited. When the energy reserves are depleted, the stage of exhaustion ensues which often ends in a terminal illness.

In my previous study, *Bioenergetics*, I pointed out that the main function of the adrenal glands is the mobilization of the body's reserve energy to cope with stress or distress. Adrenaline from the medulla of the gland has a quick-acting effect. The corticoid hormones from the cortex have a slower but more sustained action.

In this study I am interested primarily in emotional stress and how such stress leads to distress and illness. The question that naturally arises is: In what ways does emotional stress differ from physical stress? An emotional stress acts like a physical one in its effect upon the body in that it makes a demand which requires the expenditure of energy. One difference that I can see is that the amount of emotional stress in a given situation cannot be quantified. Yet studies have been made of the relationship between life changes and illness which suggest that certain events are more powerful stressor agents than others and more likely to produce illness. I am referring to studies by Thomas H. Holmes reported in *Psychosomatics*.[5] On the basis of these studies, a table of life changes was constructed according to the magnitude of the change. The table contains 43 life changes ranging from the death of a spouse at 100 units, being fired at work (42), to Christmas at 12 units and traffic tickets at 11. The author says that "A variety of illnesses were noted to coincide with high life-change magnitude." And, "If a person has had more than 300 life-change units in the last year and gets sick in the near future, the probability is that he or she will get diabetes, schizophrenia, a heart attack, or cancer rather than headache, mononucleosis, an anxiety reaction, or asthma."[6] Life changes can be very stressful, not only because of the emotions they evoke but largely because they demand an increased output of energy to cope with the new situation.

Holmes found that the stress of life situations was intimately connected with disease. For example, when a hay fever subject was introduced into a room with a high pollen level, he developed a mild hay fever. About 20 minutes later he was asked to talk about a home situation that was full of conflict. His hay fever became exacerbated with marked symptoms. In another case backache developed during a discussion of sensitive situations. Holmes reports, "As the interview began we saw the genesis of muscle tension as recorded by the myogram and, after a short period, the report of backache. When we changed to neutral topics, the muscle tension subsided and the pain went away."[7]

Valid as such studies are to show the direct connection between emotional stress and illness, they leave unanswered some very important questions. The magnitude of life changes is not the sole factor in producing disease. Even among people in the high range of life-change magnitude, only 80% got an illness. On the other hand, 30% of the people with low life-change scores got ill. The first question then is: Why do some people become ill while others fail to do so in similar situations? The obvious answer is that some people have a greater ability to cope with life situations which would produce a state of distress in others. Broadly speaking, the difference has to be in the amount of available energy. The second question has to do with the kind of illness people develop as a consequence of emotional stress. The backache patient doesn't develop hay fever. As Holmes observes, "The backache patient's attitude toward his situation was quite different from the weeping patient's; he wanted to run away...but could not take action; he was motionless with skeletal muscles mobilized to move."[8] I believe that an inability to cry or weep predisposes a person to sinus trouble and hay fever and that it is the patient's attitude or what we call his character structure which predisposes him to certain illnesses.

To understand how character structure adds to the stress of life we need to see stress as a "constricting or impelling force." The word is related to the Latin, *strictus*, meaning constriction. We are familiar with constrictions in bioenergetics. Every chronic muscular tension represents a constriction of the organism. These constrictions deform the body and therefore, constitute a stress for the organism. Their development is a function of superego formation and they are the somatic correlates of introjected parental commands and injunctions. Thus, the injunction, "Don't raise your hand to your parent," can become structured in the body as chronic muscular tensions in the shoulder which effectively prevent the person from fully raising his arm. Superego injunctions are part of the upbringing of every child. They are the dos and don'ts which have been impressed upon the child to such a degree that they become part of his character. "Don't cry," "Don't scream," "Don't play with yourself," "Sit still," "Pull your shoulders back," "Hold your belly in," are common demands upon a child which demand an expenditure of energy and so constitute a stress. Energy is expended in the muscular action necessary to block an impulse (restraining force) or assume a posture (compelling force).

It must be recognized, however, that the neurotic character structure does not develop out of parental demands unless these demands are accompanied by the threat of punishment explicitly stated or implied. And in most cases sufficient punishment is meted out either physically or by the withdrawal of love and contact to make the threat a reality to the child. But underlying the punishment or its threat is parental hostility which the child experiences as a threat to its survival if it does not accede to parental demands. Generally the parent is not conscious of his hostility because he rationalizes his behavior. But the child's experience of this hostility is the stressful element in the situation. The hostility may be expressed in a look, in a coldness of manner or in a physical assault. The child becomes frightened, even terrified. The experience of fear in relation to his parents is a shock to the child's organism. Terror is actually a state of shock. Let me add further that the implied threat of castration associated with the Oedipal situation is another shock to the organism.

The phenomenon of shock denotes the operation of an overwhelming stress, a trauma, which puts the body in a state of distress. The body's response is the alarm reaction of the G.A.S. But the stressful situation does not change and so the child is forced to make an adaptation in the form of superego. Its formation denotes that the child is now in the stage of resistance and no longer experiences distress. This does not mean that the stress has been eliminated. The child copes with the situation by using his will which is an emergency mechanism that mobilizes the body's energy reserves. The stress now exists in the chronic muscular tensions that deform the body.

Chronic muscular tensions serve to suppress forbidden and dangerous impulses from consciousness and expression. They are, in effect, locked up so that one need not spend conscious energy guarding against them. It is like imprisoning a dangerous criminal who can be guarded with less energy once he is behind bars. But no prison is fully escape proof. And no superego regardless of how strong can free the person from the possible danger that the suppressed impulse may break out. This impulse is an expression of the person's life force and is, therefore, constantly seeking release. Any breakdown of the defensive structure due either to additional stress or other forces can raise the possibility of such a release. That possibility may be strong enough to evoke the original fear and throw the body into a state of distress. It is this possibility that makes the discussion of emotional conflicts so stressful for many people. Shocks of this kind, if repeated or intense enough, will upset a person's adaptation, undermine his resistance and leave him open to breakdown and illness.

The immediate effect of suppressing impulses is to restrict the life of the individual. Chronic muscular tension is like a straight-jacket which limits a person's respiration and reduces his energy. At the same time he is under a cultural pressure to achieve some goal that would gain him the love he needs. Thus the person is not only restricted in his energy production but he is also subject to additional demands requiring the expenditure of energy. For most people in this situation the stress is very great. It accounts for the almost universal complaints of fatigue and tiredness. Most people do manage to keep going but by an effort of will. Inevitably, as Seyle demonstrated the stage of resistance passes into that of exhaustion. The person runs out of energy to keep going on. He becomes ill. The illness can be mild or severe. It may be a common cold or any other of the typical psychosomatic diseases such as arthritis, gastrointestinal disorders, high blood pressure, cardiovascular accidents, cancer, lupus erythematosus, migraine, etc. But the person can also develop a severe depression or go into a psychotic break if he is more disposed to mental illness. The illness generally removes the person from the original stressful situation and so can allow the person to recuperate and recover his energy. It does, of course, introduce a new stress in the form of the disease process. In the next section, I will discuss some aspects of the relationship of these illnesses to character structure and stress.

THE PSYCHOSOMATIC ILLNESSES

In this section I will present my ideas about certain illnesses which, I believe, are largely determined by stress. These are the psychosomatic illnesses so-called because there is no specific etiologic agent solely responsible for the disease. In the genesis of these illnesses emotional factors play an important role. But in a broad sense all illnesses are psychosomatic because a person's attitudes and feelings influence both the onset and course of the disease. For example, even in such a disease as tuberculosis where the etiologic agent is known, Holmes found that "in the two years prior to the onset of tuberculosis, a highly significant number of life changes was experienced by those who got the disease."[9]

The emotional and personality factors in illness have been extensively studied. *Psychosomatic Medicine* by Weiss and English has been a classic for many years. It is interesting to note that Spurgeon English was analyzed by Wilhelm Reich. Another important book on this subject is Mind and Body by Flanders Dunbar, editor-in-chief of the *Journal of Psychosomatic Medicine*. She was married to Theodore P. Wolfe, who brought Reich to the United States and translated several of his books into English. The wealth of published material on psychosomatic factors in illness is enormous. It is not my intention to review this literature. I would like to offer some new insights into these illnesses based upon an understanding of the energy process involved in the underlying stress condition. I believe it is well known that Reich was my teacher and analyst.

When I was in medical school in the years 1947-1951, 1 became interested in tuberculosis because I thought I could sense the emotional element in the disease. My interest also stemmed from my association with Wilhelm Reich and from my experiences as a Reichian therapist for two years prior to going to medical school. Tuberculosis, or consumption as it was then known, was a fairly common disease in the nineteenth century. It entered into the literary productions of that period. Thomas Mann's Magic Mountain is the best known but not the only story of life in a sanitarium. More important for our purpose is the picture of the consumptive heroine in the story, *La Dame Aux Camillias*, upon which the opera, *La Traviata* is based. In my view, the romantic longing of the heroine is associated with consumption. I see the person as being consumed by a longing that cannot possibly be fulfilled. The same element of romantic longing is found in the music of Chopin who also suffered from tuberculosis.

Why should romantic longing be associated with pulmonary tuberculosis? Longing or the desire for closeness is experienced as a flow of excitation along the front of the body which charges the mouth, lips and arms. It is the feeling that would make a child or infant reach out to its mother for contact and to nurse. The fulfillment of that desire in a child leads to bliss; but if the oral needs of the child are not satisfied, the longing persists into adulthood as an aching pain in the chest and throat. In the nineteenth century when breast feeding was common, children knew this bliss. But when they were weaned too early, the search for oral fulfillment which equals bliss becomes transformed into the search for a romantic love which cannot possibly fulfill the oral need. For an adult, fulfillment is possible only on the realistic level of sexuality as orgasm not on the romantic level of love as bliss. In the romantic individual of the nineteenth century, who was also sexually inhibited, the unfulfilled oral longing was held in the chest creating tension and imposing a stress upon the lungs. This stress predisposed the person to tuberculosis.

The emotional stress of unfulfilled oral longing is not the only causative factor in this disease. The person has to be exposed to the germ. It has long been recognized, however, that not every person exposed to the germ develops the illness. We must look, therefore, for other factors. Poor living conditions, overcrowding, inadequate nutrition, lack of fresh air and exercise, and fatigue operate to deplete a person's energy and make him unable to cope with infection. However, the person's characterological attitude is the factor that largely determines what illness he will develop if the stress of life becomes unbearable.

If tuberculosis can be considered the representative disease of the nineteenth century in part because it was related to the romanticism of that century, what disease is associated with the attitude of twentieth century individuals? When I posed this question to my friends after having described the relationship of tuberculosis to the romanticism of the past century, they immediately answered cancer. I had thought the same thing. This means that there is an emotional attitude which has the same relation to cancer that romantic longing has to tuberculosis. It would also be the typical attitude of the second half of this century. That attitude is despair. The idea that disease and culture are related is expressed by Henry E. Sigerist. He says, "In every epoch certain diseases are in the foreground and...are characteristic of this epoch and fit into its whole structure."[10]

Let me say that Wilhelm Reich had the same idea. He proposed that the terrain in which cancer developed is emotional resignation. He described the cancer process as a shrinking of the life energy in the body and the cancer cells as a product of the disintegration of normal tissue. Anyone interested in a deeper understanding of the cancer process than is offered by traditional medicine should read Reich's book, *The Carcinomatous Shrinking Biopathy*. However, despair is not the same thing as emotional resignation for despair does not exist without hope. When hope is lost or given up, despair becomes resignation which is a surrender to death. In the cancer patient these emotional attitudes are not conscious. It is characteristic of the cancer patient to deny his despair and, later, the emotional resignation in which it ends.

The denial of despair creates a situation of stress for the organism which slowly depletes its energy reserves. This is clear when we realize that the denial consists of a program of seemingly meaningful activity enveloped in a facade of optimism. The false optimism is a defense against the underlying despair and prevents its discharge in weeping and wailing. The activity, too, leads nowhere since it is unconsciously designed to deny the despair. It takes considerable energy and will power to keep the body up and moving in the face of an intense desire to give up and let go. When exhaustion finally sets in, the organism resigns itself to death and slowly surrenders its life. That is the unconscious process. On the conscious level every effort is made to maintain the facade of optimism and to carry on. It may seem like a contradiction to say that if one gives in to despair, one finds life and joy, but it is true as I explain in my new book, *The Fear of Life*. The despair stems from the experiences of childhood and represents one's helplessness to gain the love of the parents. We are equally helpless as adults to gain love but our need is more to love than to be loved. We also need to love ourselves. On that level, we are not helpless and there is no real cause for despair.

Some explanation is required for the statement that despair is the typical attitude of the second half of the twentieth century. I relate despair to the lack of love in life, not to love in the spiritual sense but to love in the bodily sense of joy and good cheer. How much joy is there in our world? We are so obsessed with power, productivity and performance that the simple pleasures of life escape us. We are driven, to use a popular advertising slogan. Or, to put it differently: we are slaves to an economic system that promises fulfillment but delivers frustration. The more progress we make up the economic ladder the less freedom we have and without freedom, there is no joy. We can be fulfilled as human beings only when our lives are rooted in our bodies, our animal nature and the earth. Unfortunately, our technological culture cuts us off more and more from these fundamental connections. I despair of ever fully establishing my connections, gaining my freedom or finding joy. But my despair is conscious and expressed. And since I don't believe in the system, I am not enslaved by it. I can experience some joy in my life.

Given the characterological attitude in my personality I am more vulnerable to a heart attack than to cancer. Myocardial infarction may also be regarded as a common disease of modern, twentieth century man. I believe that my vulnerability to this disease stems from the rigidity of my chest which creates a stress for the heart. I have known a number of men who suffered heart attacks and each one was marked by a tight, rigid thorax held in an inflated position. To understand why rigidity of the thoracic cage constitutes a stress situation for the heart, we have to understand the emotional attitude expressed by the rigidity. Like all muscular armoring, it is a defense against being hurt. The rigidity of the chest wall functions like a breast plate protecting the heart. Of course, the feared hurt is not physical but emotional. In effect the person is saying, "I'll allow no one to touch my heart." This maneuver makes sense to the person because he has suffered a deep hurt. His heart was "broken" by the lack of parental love and understanding. So he protects his poor, "broken" heart by locking it up in a rigid cage.

But the heart longs to be free and open for without freedom there is no joy and without joy there is no love. Yet the person does not dare to soften his chest and open his heart; his fear of being hurt is too great. He is therefore trapped by the very defense he erected to protect himself. And his heart is literally trapped in its cage. The stress, in this situation, is created by the desire to break out and be free and the fear of breaking out or by the desire to love and the fear of getting hurt. Caught in this conflict, the person is deeply frustrated and has a great resentment. But these feelings are not expressed because of a powerful sense of guilt stemming from the fear of love. This inner dynamic leads this individual into situations in which he feels trapped: it could be an unsatisfactory job or an unsatisfactory marriage. Unable to get free, he is vulnerable to a heart attack.

In my opinion the heart attack follows a reaction of panic in the individual. The panic is not experienced as such before the heart attack; rather, the myocardial infarction itself is experienced as panic. One might think, therefore, that the heart attack is the cause of the feeling of panic, but this view overlooks the fact that panic is the emotional attitude of persons who develop heart attacks. That panic is expressed in the rigid, over-inflated chest, and is the feeling of being trapped. Although we say "I feel trapped," it is more accurate to say "I feel panic because I sense that I am trapped." However, the rigidity of the chest wall which constitutes the trap and creates the state of panic is at the same time a defense against the perception of the panic. The armoring negates the person's vulnerability and panic while it expresses both.

Most persons who become ill are not aware of the forces in their personality which predispose them to illness. This lack of awareness allows the stress to build to the breaking point. The potential heart attack victim does not sense that he is trapped nor the panic associated with it. He may and often does take special measures to suppress this awareness. The most common means is the abuse of alcohol. This was illustrated by the case of a man who, after returning home in the evening from a high pressure job in the city, had several drinks before dinner following which he watched television until he fell asleep; a pattern he repeated almost every working day. It was the behavior of a trapped man who could not face his life situation. One morning on his way to his office he dropped dead of a heart attack.

If we can recognize in some individuals a predisposing cause of heart attacks, we can only guess at the precipitating cause. What happens to set off the coronary closure which causes the heart attack? Why does it occur at one moment and not another? Why this day and not an earlier one? We can answer that prior to the attack the person is in the stage of resistance or adaptation. He is coping, so it seems, with the stress. When an organism is in the stage of adaptation or resistance, it means that the stress has been overwhelming and that coping was achieved by mobilizing the reserve energy and the will. The nature of the stress that leads to CHD (coronary heart disease) was intensively studied by Rosenman and Friedman. That stress according to these authors resides in a situation in which a challenge to achieve or accomplish is accepted by an individual who "exhibits enhanced personality traits of aggressiveness, ambitiousness, competitive drive, is work-oriented with preoccupation with deadlines, and exhibits impatience and a strong sense of time urgency." Persons showing these traits are called Type A individuals. They frequently have high blood pressure and elevated blood cholesterol levels. The high blood pressure reflects a high intensity drive which is maintained by a rigidification of the arteries. The arteries, including the coronary arteries, of these individuals become more and more atherosclerotic. This hardening of the arteries which is associated with a narrowing of their lumen is the product of the stress these persons are under. The stage of adaptation is limited time-wise, as we know, by the available reserve energy and when that is used up, a breakdown must occur. This is a quantitative factor which operates in all illness.

The diagnosis of Type A individuals is most easily made by the person's physical characteristics according to Rosenman and Friedman. Some of these are an overall state of body tension (lack of body relaxations, upper chest breathing, taut facial musculature, explosive and hurried speech patterns, brisk and impatient body movements, etc.). These bodily signs express a degree of pain as well as drive. The sense of urgency also reflects an underlying panic. In fact the drive of the Type A individual is motivated by an unconscious panic. He is driven to break out or break free because on some level he feels trapped. There is no joy in the life of the competitive person and, by implication, no freedom. By the same token he has neither the time nor the energy for love. To my great surprise I found the following statement in a fortune cookie: "Love is a softening of the hearteries."

In addition to the predisposing effect of continuous stress, CHD is often precipitated by a new emotional shock which adds an extra burden of stress to an already over-burdened organism. In the case of heart attack, the new shock may be the failure of an attempt to break free from the trap. Strangely, it is just the attempt to break free which evokes the panic as an active force. I have seen this happen often in therapy where, hopefully, the person is prepared for such a development. The breakdown of the defensive position allows the suppressed feelings to emerge. If the defense is based upon a rigid chest wall, mobilizing the chest through deep breathing can evoke the underlying panic. This happened to me in my first therapeutic session with Reich which I described in *Bioenergetics*. The attempted break out can take the form of a new move, a surge of feeling or an exciting thought. If the person can't handle the ensuing anxiety or panic, he will close down the opening. Something like this occurs during the heart attack which is a closing down of an artery in the heart which may cause a closing of the heart itself.

In most cases of CHD the closing down of a coronary artery is due to spasm which is often superimposed upon arteriosclerotic or hardened arteries. Only recently have doctors become aware of the important role that spasm plays in heart attacks. Arterial spasm is a function of the adrenergic or sympathetic nervous system which is activated by cold, stress or strong emotion. Reich identified the sympathetic nervous system with anxiety while its opposite number, the parasympathetic system, is identified with pleasure. The latter system dilates arteries. The picture is fairly clear. Coronary spasm results from an anxiety attack in the heart. The anxiety or pain arises from a deep-seated sense of being trapped. Finally we must recognize that spasm is the muscle's response to shock.

The above ideas grew out of my observation of several men whom I knew well who had heart attacks. Two of the cases were instructive. These were men whose first marriages ended in divorce and who remarried shortly afterward. The new relationship developed, however, after the divorce. The first marriage had been unsatisfactory and they had gotten out. But the second proved equally unsatisfactory and both men felt trapped. One of them made an effort to change his life, to realize more pleasure and fulfillment but just as this effort might have come to some fruition, he had a heart attack and gave it up. Not one of these men was prepared to face the fact of being trapped or to deal openly and directly with his feelings.

The best protection against heart attacks is love. The heart that loves is free and joyful. But for the love to be fully effective as a prevention it has to be expressed physically. The most intense physical expression of love is the sexual orgasm. In the full orgasm the heart is released from its cage since the boundaries of the self are eliminated. The ecstasy of the orgasm is tied to this great sense of freedom. After a good orgasm one feels his heart to be light and joyful. All the tension surrounding it seems to have disappeared. One feels rejuvenated; one's heart is young again. Such an orgasm is only possible if one is free to love fully.

Arthritis is another illness that can only be understood as a reaction to stress. This statement is based on the facts that no germ has been implicated as the etiological agent and that cortisone, an anti-stress medication, is effective in treating the symptoms. Cortisone acts by suppressing the inflammatory process in the joints which Seyle sees as a maladaptation, an over-reaction of the body to "comparatively innocuous injuries."[11]

Over-reaction by the body to "comparatively innocuous injuries" is seen in allergies. Anyone who has suffered from hay fever knows how violently the body can react to a minor irritant which pollen is. But pollen is only the precipitating cause whose action is similar to the match that lights the fuse. The explosive substance is the predisposing cause. In the case of hay fever this is the hypersensitivity of the tissues which is due to the continuing stress they are under. That stress is caused by the suppression of crying which occurred because of shock. A parent's angry tones ordering a child to stop crying can come as a shock to the organism. This shock will lead to a conflict between the need to cry and the fear of crying. If this conflict is active at the time pollen is in the air, the tissues will become sensitized to it. But to understand the hay fever reaction we must see it as an attempt to discharge the underlying tension and not as a simple response to the irritant. As long as the conflict is alive, pollen will be able to set off the hay fever reaction. Antihistamines prevent the hay fever reaction by drying out the mucous membranes and so de-activating the conflict by deadening the tissues.

People overreact constantly to any situation which recalls a previous trauma or conflict. This is constantly seen in bioenergetic therapy. The best example is the person's reaction to any pressure on the tense muscles surrounding the genital organs. Many patients jump almost out of their skins when this is done. They react with shock out of fear of being injured there. This fear is their castration anxiety which they developed in the Oedipal period when they felt that they were threatened with castration for competing sexually with the parent of the same sex. That early experience came as a real shock to the organism and caused the withdrawal of sexual feeling or energy from the pelvis.[12] Some energy returns after the shock subsides but it is tentative and rigorously controlled. Any unexpected move that I make with my fingers while working in that area often produces a shock-like reaction in the patient. Obviously it recalls the earlier experience and evokes the same response. Similarly a child who has been bitten by a dog can become hysterical at the approach of a strange dog.

The weakness in Seyle's understanding of arthritis is that he fails to appreciate the power of emotional factors in producing distress and disease. The experiments of Harold G. Wolfe and his associates at New York Hospital have clearly demonstrated that simply discussing emotionally painful subjects with patients produces an exacerbation of their difficulties. The following is an example: "Where persons both normotensive and hypertensive were subjected to interviews arousing personal conflicts with conscious or unconscious anxiety and resentment there occurred in association with the elevated arterial pressure shortening of the clotting time and sedimentation rate and an increase in blood viscosity."[13] This kind of response to stress was found in most other sensitive organ systems. Thus, in a patient with an exposed colon, an increased vascularity, motility and fragility of the mucosa was noted when a discussion about his sister-in-law activated feelings of hostility, resentment and guilt.

These two examples from Wolfe's study show the immediate distressful effect of emotional conflict. But the question that few investigators can answer clearly is: Why does one person react to stress with arthritis while another develops ulcerative colitis? They are agreed that organ vulnerability is determined by early life experiences which create patterns of behavior in dealing with stress. What, then, is the pattern of behavior that predisposes an individual to arthritis? Let us examine the arthritic problem bioenergetically.

Arthritis is a disturbance of the motility of an organism. The arthritic joint is literally frozen due either to the pain of the inflammatory process or to degenerative processes in the articular surfaces. But the inflammation and the degeneration are both secondary phenomena. The disturbance in motility actually precedes the arthritic condition. We know from our study of persons with this condition that they have in their personality a strong conflict about the expression of aggressive impulses. This conflict is just under the surface in contrast to masochistic individuals where it is more deeply suppressed. The arthritic person tends to have a rigid character structure although masochistic tendencies are present. There may even be a marked schizoid element in the personality. It is the rigidity which predisposes the person to arthritis. For example, in hands which have some arthritis, one finds a tendency for contracture in flexion of the fingers. The arthritic hand in its contracted state often resembles a claw. One can surmise that the unconscious blocking of the impulse to claw is what creates the contraction.

In a case where the arthritis in the hands was very severe resulting in a pronounced claw-like malformation, I suggested to the person that her condition may be due to suppressed aggressive impulses. The suggestion was vehemently rejected. This person was an artist and saw herself as sensitive and considerate. Her ego image would not admit the possibility that she could harbor hostile or negative aggressive impulses. But since such impulses exist in all persons in our culture, her denial betrayed the conflict. The need to suppress them imposes a considerable stress upon the body. However, as long as one has the energy to meet the stress, the person is in a state of resistance and symptoms of the illness do not develop. Energy depletion or additional stress in the form of a shock could throw the organism into the illness.

When the expression of feeling meets a strong hostile response from the environment the organism is thrown into a state of shock. Children are constantly being shocked by the negative responses of their parents. As we have seen the shock is due to the withdrawal of energy from the surface of the body. The effect of shock is to freeze the body into immobility. This shock is similar to that which produces the schizoid condition. In the latter case, the shock is more severe and more prolonged and results from a denial of the child's right to be. The schizoid personality is, therefore, locked into a state of frozen immobility. When the parents are less hostile and the shock in consequence is less severe, there is an energetic rebound which overcomes the frozen state. Some aggressivity is restored but the child soon learns to be careful not to antagonize his parents. He develops control over the expression of negative feelings through the formation of a superego. This control is manifested on the body level in the form of muscular tension and rigidity. The child has made a seemingly successful adaptation and the situation has become stabilized. The stress is still operative on an unconscious level. The organism is in the stage of resistance.

The arthritic attack generally develops following one or more shocks in response to some aggressive impulses. The shock need not and often does not result from some outside action. The person becomes frightened by his own aggressive feelings and unconsciously withdraws his energy from his limbs, which are his aggressive organs. The withdrawal of energy from the periphery of the body is generally followed by a resurgence of energy. This rebound or flow of energy back into the frozen joint produces the inflammation characteristic of rheumatoid arthritis and the associated pain. Such a sequence of events is in line with our basic concept that the illness represents the body's attempt to regain its full functional capacity.

Adele Davis, the famous nutritionist, who had been in Reichian therapy, tells the story of a woman who consulted her about an arthritic condition in her hands and elbows. In talking to the patient, Davis realized that the woman had a great anger towards her brother. Davis produced a pillow and had the woman beat the pillow with her fists to vent the anger. Immediately following this expression of anger, the woman's hands and elbows felt free from pain and in a short time the arthritic condition cleared up.

I have worked with a number of arthritic patients and I must confess that I have not had a similar result. I have not been able to get any of them to fully express their anger. My attempts to have them do so have generally resulted in a worsening of the arthritic condition. And, consequently, they stopped the therapy. My failure was due to the fact that I never got them to express any real anger because they were too frightened or felt too guilty. So instead of getting the energy through into their hands and limbs, they withdrew energy leading to shock and an exacerbation of their illness. I have come to the conclusion that in the future I would require the patient to confront his fear and guilt about his hostility before getting him to express anger.

Let us now look at ulcerative colitis. Wolfe who studied some of these patients says, "The patient with ulcerative colitis is characteristically an outwardly calm, superficially peaceful individual of more than usual dependence. On going beneath this calm exterior it becomes apparent that this outwardly placid person is 'sitting on a powder keg' of intense hostility, resentment and guilt."[14] But this description also fits many arthritic patients and even others who do not react with physical symptoms. We need to know why the attack strikes one person in the gut, another in the joints, and a third elsewhere. In part this answer can be supplied by an analysis of the patient's background. But another part of the answer must be derived from an analysis of the dynamics of the illness.

The withdrawal of energy from the lower gut is associated with the emotion of fear. The basis for this statement is the language of the body. In this language "to have guts" is to have courage. However, since everyone has "guts," the expression makes sense only if it refers to the feeling of the guts. A person who feels his guts has courage, the person who doesn't is a coward, that is, frightened. Sensing or sensation is a function of the energetic charge. Thus, when a person is very frightened, "scared shitless," as the expression goes, energy is withdrawn from the guts. This constitutes a state of shock in the abdomen. The rebound or return of energy and blood produces the bloody diarrhea of ulcerative colitis. This reaction is due to the fact that the "shocked" state of the mucous lining of the gut cannot hold the returning charged fluid which then pours into the colon together with the sloughed-off lining of the gut. In less severe cases, the result is a mucous colitis. When the stress or fear is more severe, ulceration occurs in the gut as Seyle observed and there is bleeding into the intestine.

Although fear affects the gut in every individual, not everyone reacts with colitis. In many persons the target area of fear is the eyes. We say, "His eyes went wide with fear." A person is predisposed to this reaction by the experiences of early childhood. I believe that when the reaction is in the gut, it is related to a lack of support. The feeling of being helpless in the face of what seems like an overwhelming threat is the fear that shocks the gut. Infants and very young children experience this kind of fear when they become frightened by a strange person or sound in the absence of a mother or parent. Individuals who are emotionally fixated on this early level are predisposed to this kind of reaction. Such persons can be described as having an oral character which denotes a lack of nurture and support from the mother figure. And such persons, as Wolfe pointed out, are more than usually dependent.

The stress in these individuals is not caused by the dependency but by the effort to deny the need for support. This is done by tightening the belly and the guts so that one doesn't feel anxious or insecure. One doesn't feel secure by this maneuver, rather it is a maneuver to cut off sensation. In effect the person is holding himself up by his guts. In the oral character, as I pointed out in The Language of the Body, the legs are weak but held rigidly. The rigidity provides an illusion of "standing on one's own feet" while in reality, the oral character clings to others. As in other illnesses, the disease does not surface until the person enters the stage of exhaustion. Prior to that time the oral character is in the stage of resistance. By using his reserve energy he can cope with the stress created by the denial and suppression of his insecurity and need. But another shock stemming from danger together with the feeling of helplessness or the withdrawal of support by a loved person can result in an attack of ulcerative colitis. The situation then becomes more than the person can handle and he is in a state of distress.

Because of the early deprivation of love and support the oral character harbors strong feelings of resentment and hostility. And since these feelings are directed mainly at the person in the nurturing position, they are accompanied by guilt. "Don't bite the hand that feeds you," is a saying that would make a child feel guilty for his hostility towards the mother. Actually the feeling of hostility is suppressed in the interest of survival long before the superego develops. The suppression of hostility provides the somatic basis for the idea of guilt.

If the above analysis is correct, the treatment of this condition must aim at helping the person gain an inner sense of support which would derive from fully feeling one's legs on the ground. This requires a program of intensive physical work with the legs and feet to bring the energy and feeling into them. But such a program will be resisted by the patient with this illness. Like any oral character he has no confidence that the ground will be there for him any more than his mother was. The mother is the baby's first "ground" and remains forever identified with the earth and the ground. And so the patient will not dare to fall. The fear of falling is related to the fear of being helpless and abandoned. To counter the fear of falling one tenses the leg muscles turning them into rigid supports which lack feeling. At the same time the person tightens his gut not to feel scared. The intensive physical work with the legs is not designed to make the legs harder but softer. As a result of the exercises the person's legs will feel weaker not stronger. He will feel that his legs won't hold him up. This feeling is the true perception of his legs and denotes that he is now in touch with them and with the ground. It denotes also that the rigidity has greatly diminished. There is anxiety in the feeling that one's legs won't hold one up. It is called falling anxiety. Then as one passes through this anxiety by continuing to work with the legs, they become stronger because they can support the person without becoming rigid.

At the same time, one works with the person's breathing to make it deeper, more abdominal. And one will also work directly on the tense muscles of the gut and abdominal wall to get them relaxed. This work will lead to crying in the form of deep sobs. With the release of this crying the gut becomes relaxed. And it will stay relaxed if the emotional conflicts buried in the personality are analyzed and worked through.

I believe this approach would be effective in curing a person of ulcerative colitis. However, like all neurotic individuals, he will offer some resistance to the process of getting well. In part this resistance stems from the fear which underlies the condition and which the person is reluctant to experience. Unconsciously, he will make every effort to avoid feeling the weakness of his legs and the associated falling anxiety. That is his neurotic pattern. Another source of the resistance is the secondary gains the person derives from being ill. As a sick person he doesn't have to stand on his own legs really and he will also get the support and attention he longed for. Once one is sick it becomes an easy way out in the sense that one can give up the neurotic struggle to overcome one's weaknesses without admitting that one has failed.

In a deeper sense the illness offers the person a real chance to work out his neurotic attitudes and find a healthier way to live. The breakdown into illness stops the neurotic struggle which has exhausted the person's energy and may allow, in the phase of convalescence, a rebuilding of energy reserves. From this point of view all illness can be seen as the body's attempt to get well. Everything depends on whether the person can understand and go along with his body's feelings rather than fighting to control them.

PREVENTING ILLNESS—COPING WITH STRESS

We have said that stress results from a situation which makes a demand upon the organism for the expenditure of energy. If the organism has sufficient energy to meet the demand, there is no problem. Trouble arises when the demand is excessive. In that case the normal and healthy response is to withdraw from the situation. All animals follow this pattern of behavior which is directed by the pleasure/pain principle. We experience the process of living as pleasurable when we have sufficient energy to meet the demands of life. When the demand is excessive or we are deficient in energy, the stress becomes distress which is painful. The pleasure/pain principle says that all organisms seek pleasure and try to avoid pain.

Human beings are also governed by another principle called the reality principle. This says that a person will forego pleasure and tolerate pain if he believes that such behavior will lead to a greater pleasure or to the avoidance of a greater pain in the future. Because of this principle known as reality people do not always withdraw from distressing or painful situations. A young child faced with a hostile and punishing parent cannot physically withdraw from the situation. Being alone is more frightening than the pain he must endure. But his submission does not relieve the shock effect of the hostility or punishment.

There is an alternative to flight. If one has the energy and strength, one can fight the aggressor which, if successful, may prevent the pain and the distress. Fight or flight are the basic animal responses to distressing or painful situations. In both fight and flight the energy reserves of the organism are mobilized through the action of adrenaline to meet the emergency. Such emergencies in the animal world are generally of short duration—an attack by a predator, for example. The prey escapes and the emergency ends.

Generally, there is no escape from parental hostility. The child is forced to submit to the demands of his parents. On a physical level he can neither flee nor fight but he can do one or both psychologically.

He can withdraw psychologically from a situation by cutting his contact with reality. This is done by withdrawing energy from the periphery of the body. It is the schizoid or schizophrenic pattern and it is also the equivalent of shock. The schizophrenic individual is in a more or less permanent state of shock which numbs him to reality. So in that state the stress of life or of reality does not affect him and he will not develop a psychosomatic illness as described above. Autopsies of schizophrenics have shown that their heart and blood vessels are like those of young people. The price he pays for this protection from stress is the withdrawal from life. He exists in a state of limbo, neither dead nor fully alive. By withdrawing he limits his ability to take in energy, his breathing is very shallow. I mentioned earlier that the schizophrenic individual is not as susceptible to colds as others because he remains in a somewhat frozen condition. However, because of his poor respiration he is liable to pneumonia as he gets older. In the past before antibiotics this was often his fatal illness.

Psychologically one fights by tensing the body so that one can take the punishment without breaking down. On the surface the child seems to have submitted; internally, he stiffens to resist the parents' demands. This tensing and stiffening of the muscles may be localized or generalized but in both cases he says "I won't" in the language of the body. But by this maneuver the conflict becomes internalized since by his overt submission the child's ego incorporates the parents' demands as valid goals. Thus one part of the ego, the superego or ego ideal, commands the fulfillment of these goals while another part, the suppressed resistance, fights against their attainment. The child also accepts the parents' rationalization and justification for their negative attitude—namely, that if the child was as the parents wished, he would be loved. This is the typical pattern of the neurotic individual who accepts the reality as his parents proclaim it and strives to fulfill their demands. He will be as his parents demanded. But all he can really do is erect a facade of conformity since inwardly he is just the opposite.

The basic difference between the schizophrenic and the neurotic attitude is that whereas the former represents a withdrawal of energy from the surface and reality, the latter is based on an overinvestment in the surface appearance as the true reality. Thus, we saw that the person who suffers from ulcerative colitis, the oral character type, has created a facade which denies his needing, his dependency and his fear of falling. The person who develops arthritis, basically a rigid type, denies his negative aggressivity and presents a facade of care and solicitude for others. Recently I worked with a young woman who suffered from lupus erythematosus. This is an illness which may properly be described as self-destructive in that part of the body, the immune system, seems to react negatively to its own tissues. The symptoms in her case were weakness, pulmonary inflammation, a facial outbreak, and eye disorders. Her facade was that of being "daddy's good little girl." This role required an inhibition of her sexuality, a suppression of her romantic longing and a denial of her rage at her father and men. In return she expected love and protection from her father and other men with whom she became involved. She had never gotten this from her father nor from any man. She did get implied promises of love and protection that were never fulfilled. Yet she believed in them and invested her energy into the effort to make them into reality.

As long as she could maintain the facade she was in the stage of resistance and free from any symptoms of disease. She was, however, under great stress because maintaining the facade imposed much self-denial, and demanded considerable energy. She was close to the stage of exhaustion. And then, she had a shock. She was betrayed by a man who was in the position of a father surrogate. Judging by her reaction it was a severe shock for one day later she was in the hospital with a high fever. Cortisone slowly brought her condition under control and her symptoms disappeared but further stress reactivated them.

In therapy with me she made some progress—feeling stronger and better. As her therapist I became a father surrogate who was supposed to protect and love her. In return she would be my little girl. Being a therapist involves much more than being loving and protecting to patients: I had to take a hard look at the patient's neurotic attitude and confront her with it. When I did this my patient felt betrayed and her symptoms reappeared in milder form. It was another shock. When I was away for the summer, her anger at me brought a recrudescence of her eye symptoms. And yet only through such shocks and the return of the illness could she discern the pattern that made her liable to this disease.

The maintenance of a facade predisposes a person to somatic illness because it imposes a constant stress upon the body. One tries to be what one isn't which deforms the personality and the body. When the deformation (stress) persists long enough, the internal structure of the body breaks down. It is not the facade that breaks down but the tissues of the body. The facade is maintained even at the cost of structural integrity. In the case of schizophrenia, it is the surface of the personality that breaks down under overwhelming stress while the internal organs are protected. We can put it another way. In schizophrenia the breakdown is mental or psychic whereas in the neuroses it is physical or somatic. This is clearly seen in the case of cancer.

I have related cancer to despair. The cancer victim almost never acknowledges his despair. He maintains a facade of courage and hope almost to the very end. He dies on the inside while maintaining a facade of interest in life on the surface. The schizophrenic, on the other hand, is never far from his despair. He cannot handle it any better than the cancer patient but he does not attempt to overcome it. By his withdrawal, he dies on the outside while guarding a core of integrity on the inside.

I am not trying to say that mental illness is better or worse than somatic illness. Neither is health which is what we want. I have written extensively about the problems of mental illness elsewhere. Here, I would like to focus on the psychosomatic illnesses and the problem of undue stress. But we need to know the energy dynamics that underlie these illnesses if we wish to treat them or prevent them.

The Voice of the Body

We all know that the life style of modern society creates enormous stress for its members. The demands upon them are great and, often, excessive. These demands are, broadly speaking, to produce, to achieve, and to accomplish. The goals are success, power and fame. The attainment of these goals requires that the person devote almost all his energy to this task. This is especially true since the culture is also very competitive. People who are committed to the goals of this culture have no place in their lives for feelings. The drive for success requires the development of a rigid personality structure based on the suppression of all feeling including sexuality. The person becomes a doer, an achiever, a performer. In most families the training for this life style starts early in the life of the child.

The suppression of feeling is done by muscular contraction which places the body in a state of tension. While the tension creates the drive, it also reduces the body's energy through its restriction of respiration. The result is that persons who drive themselves are heading for a breakdown. This analysis suggests only one way to avoid illness and that is by reversing the pattern of this culture. The drive or push to succeed must be reduced and the life of the body expressed through feeling must be increased. We must realize that the drive for success is an attempt to compensate for an inner sense of failure as a man or woman. It is an effort to convince our parents and the world that we are worth being loved despite the fact that we don't feel lovable. But no matter how much we try nor how successful we become we never arrive at feeling loving or lovable and we succumb to the despair we refuse to acknowledge.

The key to health is to live fully the life of the body. This means that feeling is more important than doing, that being free is more important than being rich, and that the present is always more important than the future. This is not to deny some validity to the reality principle. But in sacrificing the present for the future we must be sure that the promise of future gain is not an impossible dream, an illusion that can never be fulfilled. In terms of the body there is neither success nor failure. Life is to be lived and in the living of it one grows old and dies. But when the living is postponed until success is achieved, "He made it," the end is always tragic.

Living the life of the body means being in touch with one's feelings and being able to express them. This requires that the body be free as much as possible from the chronic muscular tensions that affect all of us. We have to sense what goes on in our bodies. We can only do that if we take time to work with our bodies so that we can feel our legs and the ground, be aware of how we hold ourselves, and how we breathe. For me this means a regular program of bioenergetic exercises the rest of my life. Such a program can greatly help in keeping my energy at an optimum level.

It is most important in dealing with situations that create undue stress to have the courage to withdraw physically. We are afraid to withdraw because it feels like defeat. We hang in because not to do so is viewed as failure. We must use our wills to overcome our seeming fears and weaknesses to prove our worth. We struggle against a fate that becomes more inevitable the harder we try to avoid it. Really, we create the stressful conditions that break us down in the long run.

Notes

1. Wolfe, Harold G., *Stress and Disease*, Charles C. Thomas, Springfield, Ill., 1953, p. 4.

2. Seyle, Hans, *The Stress of Life*, McGraw-Hill, New York, 1956, p. 54.

3. Seyle, Hans, *Stress Without Distress*, New American Library, New York, 1975.

4. Ibid., p. 14.

5. Holmes, Thomas H., Life Situations, Emotions and Disease, *Psychosomatics*, Vol. 19, No. 12, Dec. 1979, pp. 747-754.

6. Ibid., p. 753.

7. Ibid., p. 748.

8. Ibid., p. 748.

9. Ibid., p. 753.

10. Sigerist, Henry E., as quoted in H. G. Wolfe, *Stress and Disease*, op. cit., p. 2.

11. Seyle, Hans, *The Stress of Life*, op. cit., p. 165.

12. See my new book, *The Fear of Life*, for a full discussion of castration anxiety.

13. Wolfe, Harold G., *Stress and Disease*, op. cit., p. 86.

14. Ibid., p. 52.

2

The Rhythm of Life
A Discussion of the Relation between Pleasure and the Rhythmic Activities of the Body

LECTURE 1: PLEASURE AND PAIN

The Mystery of Pleasure

The effort to understand the human dilemma leads inevitably to the mystery of pleasure. Since the popularization of psychoanalysis, we have accepted Freud's statement that the organism strives for pleasure and to avoid pain. Before Freud, Leslie Stephen had said, "I repeat that pain and pleasure are, according to me, the determining causes of action. It may even be said that they are the sole and ultimate causes." But while we know what pain is and can measure it objectively, the phenomenon of pleasure evades scientific observation.

Pain seems to have a substantial quality. Its severity is often directly related to the intensity of the noxious agent. A second degree burn is invariably more painful than a first degree burn. Pain is fairly consistent in that a given painful stimulus affects most people alike. And pain tends to be localized. The body contains specific pain receptors and nerves which serve to locate the source of the pain. If these nerves are blocked by an anesthetic agent, the pain disappears.

In contrast, pleasure seems to be insubstantial. If a good steak can excite our palates, two good steaks can give us indigestion. It often happens that a dinner we enjoyed yesterday is unexciting when served again today. Pleasure depends greatly upon one's mood. When we are feeling blue, the best company can be a disturbance. It is as difficult to enjoy a thing of beauty when one is depressed as it is hard to smell a rose when one has a cold. But a good mood, while indispensable to enjoyment, is not a guaranty of pleasure. On too many occasions I have gone to the theatre and cinema with keen anticipation and high spirits only to emerge deflated and denied. Pleasure seems to require a concurrence between the inner state and the outer situation.

The differences between our reactions to pain and pleasure can be explained, in part at least, by the fact that pain is a danger signal. It denotes a threat to the integrity of the organism and calls forth a mobilization of resources on an emergency basis. All senses are alerted and the musculature is readied for action. To meet the threat, the exact location of the danger must be known, its intensity gauged and all activities suspended until safety is assured.

Pleasure is elusive. The harder you look for it, the less likely you are to find it. If you grasp it too greedily, it disappears in your grip. Robert Burns writes:

> But pleasures are like poppies spread
> You seize the flower, its bloom is shed

On the other hand, it may appear in the most unexpected places; a flower that grows by the wayside, a conversation with a stranger, an unwelcome social evening that turns out to be a delightful soiree.

Pleasure cannot be possessed. One must give oneself over to pleasure, that is, let the pleasure take possession of one's being.

Pleasure is as shy as it is elusive. It hides its fair face from the vulgar regard. It abides in the lover's intimacy and vanishes when that intimacy is violated. It will not respond to command nor perform on order. Like a little girl who will hide her talents when company is present, it is the product of spontaneity. Yet pleasure is not secretive, it demands to be shared. It blossoms in the company of initiates, sympaticos and well-wishers. As everyone knows, a pleasure shared is a pleasure gained. A pleasure hidden is a pleasure lost.

As gentle as a summer breeze, as fragile as a whisper in the night, pleasure has the power to change destinies and the force to create life. It can be destroyed as easily as one can crush a flower and like the flower, it springs anew from the abundant earth. It comes unbidden, a gift of the gods, to lift up man's spirits and brighten his world. Its presence stops all inquiry; it is that which has all meaning within itself. Its absence forces man to make the search that is doomed from the start to fail.

The Nature of Pleasure

It is common knowledge that pleasure results from the satisfaction of needs. To eat when one is hungry and to sleep when one is sleepy are pleasurable experiences which illustrate this principle. Freud stated that pleasure results from the discharge of tension and postulated that the amount of pleasure is related to the gradient of the discharge; the steeper the gradient, the greater the pleasure. This is certainly true for sex where the amount of pleasure is a function of the intensity of the desire and the rate of discharge. However, a view of pleasure that limits it to the discharge of tension or the satisfaction of needs, though obviously valid, is too narrow to comprehend human behavior.

People enjoy a certain amount of tension. They find pleasure in challenging situations such as competitive sports because the tension increases the excitation. The build-up of excitation is a pleasurable experience when it is associated with the prospect of release or satisfaction. In sexual activity, this intensification of excitement is called fore-pleasure in contrast to end-pleasure or the satisfaction of orgasm. When, however, the prospect of release is lacking or satisfaction is unduly postponed, desire and want become painful states. Thus both need and fulfillment are aspects of pleasure in the absence of conflict or disturbance.

Since the primary needs of the organism have to do with the maintenance of its integrity, pleasure is related to the sense of well-being that arises when this integrity is assured. In its simplest form, pleasure reflects the healthy operation of the vital process of the body. Pain, of course, denotes a breakdown or disturbance of the body's vital functions. Leslie Stephen makes the same point,

> We must suppose then, that pain and pleasure are correlatives of certain states which may be roughly regarded as the smooth and distorted working of the physical machinery and given these states, the sensations must always be present.

In its simplest meaning, pleasure is the sensation that develops from the ongoing process of life.

The ongoing process of life is more than mere survival, that is, it is more than the maintenance of the physical integrity of the organism. The ability to survive is found in many emotionally disturbed individuals who complain that they have little or no pleasure in living and feel depressed. In these cases, the processes of life have stopped going 'onward.' Life does not aim at a static equilibrium, but includes the concept of growth. That is why novelty is such an essential ingredient in pleasure. The repetition of identical experiences is boring and, in our minds, means life-negating. We use the expression "bored to death" to describe the harmful effects of a lack of excitement.

Pleasure is closely tied to the phenomenon of growth which is a vital expression of the ongoing process of life. We grow by the incorporation of the environment into our being both physically and psychologically;

and we enjoy the expansion and extension of our being: the increase of our strength, the development of motor coordination and skills, the broadening of our social relationships, and the enrichment of our minds. A healthy person literally has an "appetite" for life, for learning, for the incorporation of new experience into his being. This concept explains why youth, a period of active physical and mental growth, is closer to pleasure than age. It also explains why the pleasures of older people take a more intellectual form since this aspect of their personality is still capable of growth. Young people, as everyone knows, have a greater capacity for excitement than older people.

The mystery of pleasure is hidden in the phenomenon of excitation, the capacity of the living organism to hold and increase its state of excitation. The living organism does not change from inertness to responsiveness like a machine when the motor is started or the current turned on. There is a continuous excitation in the living organism which increases or decreases in response to stimuli proceeding from its environment. Broadly speaking, an increase of excitation leads to pleasure, a decrease to boredom or depression.

Excitatory phenomena occur in non-living nature. In physics, an electron is said to become excited when a particle of light energy, a photon, falls upon an atom. The energy is captured by the electron which moves to an outer orbit, a "more excited state." When this energy is released by the electron in the form of light, the electron returns to its former position, a less excited state. The lumination in our atmosphere is another example of excitation. As the sun rises above the horizon, its energy bombards the gaseous envelope of the earth. This energy is picked up by the atoms of the atmosphere which become excited and give off light. The fact that space is dark shows that daylight is an excitatory process in our own atmosphere produced by the sun's energy. One can regard the lumination of an electric light bulb as due to the same process. The electric current passing through the light bulb filament can be said to "excite" the electrons of the filament causing them to give off light.

Lumination is also an aspect of excitation in living organisms. We light up with pleasure, shine in a state of joy and glow with ecstasy. The radiance of the alive person is most clearly seen in his eyes but is also manifested in the brightness of his skin. I recall a remark made by my son when his mother commented that he did not smile when his school picture was taken. "But, Mom," he said, "see how my eyes are shining." Intense pleasure, such as full sexual orgasm, produces a sensation in the body which is directly perceived as a glow. Finally, the radiance of a person in love makes us directly aware of his happiness.

The excitation in a living organism differs from that in nature because it is contained within a closed system. The body is surrounded by a skin that acts both as a shield to protect the organism against external forces and as an envelope to hold its inner charge. Under the skin are the voluntary muscles which sheathe the body and form part of this envelope.

Individuals vary in their capacity to become excited and in their ability to contain the excitation. Some people are glum, too serious and constrained. In the theatrical world they are called "heavies." Nothing seems to excite them. Others are overexcitable, high-strung, restless and hyperactive. They cannot hold their excitation and tend to yield to every impulse.

Because it is a closed system containing an inner charge or excitation, the living body has an inherent motility. It is in constant motion, awake or asleep. The heart beats, the blood flows, the lungs expand and contract, digestion is a continuous process, etc. It moves independently through space. In man, many of these movements are conscious and ego directed, many more are involuntary movements of which he may or may not be conscious. Involuntary responses to a stimulus or situation are described as spontaneous if made consciously. A high degree of motility and spontaneity characterizes the healthy person. Both are decreased in depressed individuals.

These considerations show the intimate connection between the ongoing process of life, excitation, motion and pleasure.

Life (energy process) > Excitation > Motion > Pleasure

They are directly visible in the child who literally jumps for joy.

Pleasure can be defined as the perception or sensation of the spontaneous movements of the body. This is not to say that voluntary or ego directed movements are not pleasurable. There is an element of spontaneity in many of our conscious activities which adds pleasure to their performance. On the other hand, there is little pleasure in activities which are forced upon us or which we impose upon ourselves against our wishes or natural inclinations. Spontaneity is the heart of pleasure and joy.

The above definition, however, ignores the fact that many spontaneous or involuntary movements reflect pain rather than pleasure. The spontaneous response to a feeling of panic is unpleasant. A child in a temper tantrum is moving involuntarily but the experience is not a pleasurable one. It must be recognized that a state of excitation can be painful or pleasurable; in either case it will manifest itself in certain involuntary movements which enable the observer to distinguish one from the other.

An analysis of the movements underlying the different sensations in the pain-pleasure spectrum will reveal the nature of pleasure.

Agony•Pain•Distress•Good Feelings•Pleasure•Joy•Ecstasy

Agony may be considered the extreme form of painful sensations. Agony denotes that a painful condition has persisted beyond the endurance of the organism. In agony, the body twists and contorts in a series of convulsive movements. The final agony of death is such a convulsion.

Pain is expressed by writhing and jerking movements less convulsive than those of agony. The difference, however, is only one of degree.

Distress is a milder form of painful agitation. The body may wriggle or squirm with distress but the movements are not so spasmodic as in the above states.

Good Feelings denote a state of ease and relaxation in the body manifested in quiet and harmonious movements. This is the basic pleasure state expressed in the remark, "I feel good."

Pleasure. As the excitement mounts to pleasure, joy and ecstasy, the movements become more intense and quicker, maintaining their coordination and rhythm. In pleasure, the person feels soft, vibrant and buoyant; the eyes glow and the skin is warm. It can be said that the body purrs with pleasure.

Joy denotes an increased pleasurable excitement such that the body seems to dance. Its movements are lively and graceful.

Ectasy. In ecstasy, the highest form of pleasurable excitement, the currents in the body are so intense that the person is "lit up" like a star. The sensation is one of transport (from the earth to the cosmos). Ecstasy is experienced in the full sexual orgasm. The movements which accompany this feeling are described in my book, *Love and Orgasm.*

The difference between the movements on the pain and pleasure side of the spectrum is the quality of coordination or rhythmicity. In pain, the body's movements are uncoordinated and spasmodic, in pleasure these movements are smooth and rhythmical. These involuntary movements are the language of the body. From them one can determine the feelings of another person. Mothers can tell from the expression and body movements of an infant whether it is in a state of distress or pain, or whether it is comfortable or experiencing pleasure.

This analysis shows that pleasure cannot be defined as the absence of pain. For while it is true that the relief from pain produces a distinctly good feeling, it does so by restoring the body to its base state, good feelings. The pain has made us conscious of our bodies and in the short time following its release we are also conscious of the pleasure of being alive. We lose this consciousness and our pleasure too quickly under the pressure of our ego drives for success and status. Unfortunately, our common experience is, as Samuel Johnson put it, that "Life is a progression from want to want, not from enjoyment to enjoyment."

It is more logical to define pain in terms of pleasure than the other way around. Pleasure represents the healthy functioning of the body, pain denotes a disturbance in our being. Pain is, therefore, the loss of pleasure. We experience pain in this form psychologically when we say, "I am pained by your rejection of me."

Both pain and pleasure are natural responses of the body to its environment. When the relation of the organism to its environment is harmonious and positive, the feeling tone is pleasurable. Any threat to or disruption of that harmony is painful. There is no neutral state in nature and there is no natural condition in the organism that corresponds to an absence of pleasure and pain. From this point of view, an absence of feeling or the sensation of emptiness is pathological. Such a condition, troubling so many people, indicates that they have suppressed their feelings. They have become rigid, thereby suppressing all movement and all sensation.

It can be stated that rigidity or chronic muscular tension is designed to suppress painful sensations. Obviously, no one would want to suppress pleasurable feelings. When in the course of bioenergetic therapy, these tensions are resolved, it can be expected that painful memories and effects will emerge in consciousness. The ability of a patient to accept and tolerate these painful feelings will determine his capacity to experience pleasurable ones. The dictum, "No pleasure without pain," is applicable to these people.

The Loss of Pleasure
Pain: The Nervous Regulation of Response

The mammalian organism is equipped with two nervous systems to integrate and regulate its responses. One, the cerebrospinal system, coordinates the action of the voluntary muscles with the sensory input, proprioceptive and exteroceptive. It regulates muscular tone and maintains posture. To a varying degree, the movements it controls are subject to conscious control. The muscles upon which it acts are the striated, skeletal muscles of the body.

The second is the autonomic or vegetative nervous system which regulates the basic body processes such as breathing, circulation and heart action, digestion, elimination, glandular activity and pupillary response. The muscles upon which it acts are called smooth muscles because they lack the striations characteristic of the larger skeletal muscles. Its action is not under the conscious control, whence the name autonomic system. It is composed of two subdivisions known as the sympathetic and parasympathetic nerves which act antagonistically to each other. For example, the sympathetic nerves speed up the action of the heart, the parasympathetic slow it down.

Wilhelm Reich observed that "the parasympathetic (is) operative whenever there is *expansion, elongation, hypemia, turgo* and *pleasure.* Conversely, the sympathetic is found functioning wherever the organism contracts, withdraws blood from the periphery, where it shows *pallor, anxiety* or *pain.*"[1] Focusing too sharply upon the sexual function, Reich postulated an antithesis between pleasure and anxiety rather than pleasure and pain. The identity of pleasure and parasympathetic functions is clear, even if this concept is not fully accepted by physiologists. The sympathetic, however, through its innervation of the adrenal gland, mobilizes the body to meet the emergency created by pain or the threat of danger. It prepares the organism for fight or flight; in the process the senses are alerted (dilation of the pupils), the heart muscles are stimulated, blood pressure is raised and oxygen consumption is increased.

The two divisions have opposite effects upon the direction of blood flow. Parasympathetic action dilates the peripheral arterioles increasing the blood supply to the surface and producing greater surface warmth. Sympathetic action contracts these arterioles and forces the blood to the interior of the body to provide more oxygen for the vital organs and the musculature. In effect, parasympathetic action promotes an expansion of the organism and a reaching out to the environment, that is, a pleasurable response. Sympathetic action produces a contraction and withdrawal from the environment, a response to pain.

Anxiety is a form of fear, a reaction to the threat of pain. It has been produced experimentally in animals where its dynamics have been elucidated. If a laboratory animal is offered food (a pleasure stimulus) to which a painful stimulus is attached, the animal develops severe symptoms of anxiety. Unable to advance because its previous experience warns it of pain, unable to withdraw because of the attraction of pleasure, it becomes confused, shaky and anxious. The anxiety of neurotic patients must be explained similarly as a conflict between the opposing forces of pain and pleasure.

Every painful situation is an emergency situation to which a person responds by activating the sympathetic-adrenal system, sharpening all senses and mobilizing his will. A state of tension is created and the normal pleasurable movements of the body are suspended until the emergency passes. The concept of the will is set forth in *The Betrayal of the Body*. When the will is mobilized, the voluntary musculature of the body is alerted to stand by for orders from the command center, the conscious ego. This means that spontaneity is arrested. It is not generally appreciated that the normal movements of a person are largely autonomic and spontaneous, allowing the feelings of pleasure to be expressed in graceful and rhythmic movements. This changes in an emergency situation. The difference can be illustrated by a horseback rider who has been enjoying his gallop, allowing his horse great latitude in his movements. Faced with an emergency, he takes full control of the horse which responds to every command but the pleasure is gone for both the horse and its rider.

The will is antithetical to pleasure. Its mobilization to achieve even a minor goal reduces the feeling of pleasure. By its nature, every goal creates an emergency situation since it would be meaningless if it didn't pose a challenge and require an effort. To the degree that the goal is imperative, it demands a concentration of energy and a focusing of thought. The body's response to the challenge of a goal is not different from its response to any other emergency: the sympathetic adrenal system is activated to provide the extra energy for the effort. Whether the goal is physical such as competing in a race or psychological such as writing an article for a deadline, it creates a state of tension that belongs to the pain side of the spectrum. The familiar picture of the novelist at his typewriter, tense, nervous, frustrated and smoking one cigarette after another illustrates the intensity of the physical strain that can be imposed by a psychological goal.

Setting goals is a function of the reality principle which states that an individual will tolerate a pain or postpone a present pleasure for the sake of a greater pleasure in the future. Achieving a goal means that one can relax and enjoy the fruits of his labor. Such behavior is rational if the goal bears a true relation to the promise of pleasure. Unfortunately, most goals are status symbols which assume an exaggerated importance in the thinking of people. To earn the money for a boat is a valid activity for the person who delights in being on the water, but not for the person who regards the boat as a possession. In the second case, owning a boat may provide an ego satisfaction which I regard as a spurious pleasure.

For a great many people, the achievement of goals becomes the meaning of life. No sooner is one objective realized than another is proposed. Each achievement provides a momentary thrill of excitement that soon fades and necessitates a new goal: a new car, a better house, more money, etc. We have become obsessed with achievement and as a result we seem to have lost the capacity for pleasure. Struggling constantly to meet goals, living continually in a state of emergency, is it surprising that we suffer from high blood pressure, ulcers, tension and anxiety? We pride ourselves on our drive not realizing that every push requires the activation of the sympathetic-adrenal system.

Not every goal demands a postponement of immediate pleasure. We have seen that a state of tension can be pleasurable if it is associated with the prospect of release or fulfillment. The anticipation of pleasure is itself a pleasurable experience. In this situation, the necessary effort is easy and relaxed, the activity proceeds smoothly, almost effortlessly, and the body's movements are rhythmical and coordinated. Work of this kind is pleasurable. But one can work in this fashion only when there is no desperation, when the activity is as important as the goal, or when the end does not dominate the means. A preoccupation with goals and achievement characterizes people who are afraid of pleasure.

The Fear of Pleasure

The fear of pleasure seems like a contradiction. How can anyone fear that which is the opposite of pain? Yet, many people avoid pleasure, some develop acute anxiety in pleasurable situations, and others experience pain when the pleasurable excitation becomes intense. At the end of this lecture someone asked, "How do you explain the remark, 'It feels so good it hurts'?" This question reminded me of a remark a patient made, "It hurts good." It is well known that some people find pleasure in pain, a masochistic reaction that also requires explanation.

I shall discuss the masochistic reaction first. Consider the situation of a person who finds he has become stiff from being in one position too long. He finds it painful to stretch his cramped muscles, yet as he does so he experiences a good feeling as his circulation is restored. Another example is the person who squeezes a pimple to release its pressure. The procedure is painful, but as the pimple bursts and discharges its contents the feeling is one of pleasure and satisfaction. It can be said in both cases that the pleasure is in the release of the tension, and that the painful procedure was necessary to obtain the release. True, there is nothing masochistic in enduring some pain for the sake of pleasure. We all do this as part of the reality principle. If, as in the above examples, the release of tension accompanies the pain, it would appear that the person actually enjoys the pain.

The sexual masochist who obtains pleasure from being beaten is similarly motivated. He needs the pain to release the pleasure. His body is so rigid, and his buttocks are so tense that no sexual excitation can get through to the genitals. The beating, apart from its psychological meanings, relaxes his tensions by softening his muscles which allows the sexual excitation to flow. Wilhelm Reich pointed out in his study of masochism that the masochist is not interested in the pain per se, but seeks the pleasure that is released by the pain. I have further elaborated on this concept in *The Physical Dynamics of Character Structure.*

It is interesting to note that traumas are not always immediately painful. Sometimes one does not even feel the cut that is inadvertently inflicted by the slip of a sharp knife. Moments later there is a sudden pain as waves of feeling flood the injured area. The knife cut is like a shock which leaves the injured part momentarily stunned. The same thing happens with psychological traumas. An insult is often not perceived the minute it is uttered. The pain of the insult seems to strike us later as a wave of anger floods our being. It can be that the insult caught us off guard, and we are unprepared to react: but this seems to be generally true of insults.

Frostbite is the prime example of a painless trauma and a painful recovery. The person who has frostbite may be unaware of the condition until he enters a warm room. Then the pain begins, and it becomes increasingly severe as the blood flows into the frozen extremity. Obviously the freezing of the part cut off all feeling. This procedure is even used as an anesthetic. Pain, it would appear, is a response to the trauma. It is a reaction of the body to the injury, a reaction that aims to overcome the injury. It is also a warning of danger, a sign that the thawing out process must be slow to avoid any permanent loss of function.

The individual whose body is tense, tight and contracted is in a situation similar to that of frostbite. He is frozen in his immobility and lack of spontaneity. In a situation of pleasure he is exposed to a warmth produced by the flow of blood to the periphery of the body through the action of the parasympathetic nerves. The pleasure induces an expansion in his body which is momentarily painful, and may even be frightening. This body sensation is definitely not pleasurable. The person feels as if he will burst or fall apart. His immediate thought is to get out of the situation.

Were he to stay in the situation and allow the pleasure to increase, he would experience the falling apart physically. He would begin to tremble and vibrate and to feel shaky. He would feel that he has lost control over his body; his movements would be awkward; his self-possession would be lost. His body tensions and their psychological counterpart, his ego defenses, would give way. This has happened to many people in such situations. They become so nervous they are forced to withdraw. However, if the shakiness is allowed to proceed, it will end in crying. The crying is a breaking down of rigidity provoked by an overwhelming pleasure. Examples of this reaction are numerous. Many women cry following a pleasurable sex experience. People cry when they encounter long lost friends or relatives. The saying is, "I am so happy I could cry."

As adults, we have many inhibitions against crying. We feel it is an expression of weakness, or femininity or of childishness. The person who is afraid to cry is afraid of pleasure. This is because the person who is afraid to cry holds himself together rigidly so that he won't cry; that is, the rigid person is as afraid of pleasure as he is afraid to cry. In a situation of pleasure he will become anxious. As his tensions relax he will begin to tremble and shake, and he will attempt to control this trembling so as not to break down in tears. His anxiety is nothing more than the conflict between his desire to let go and his fear of letting go. This conflict will arise whenever the pleasure is strong enough to threaten his rigidity.

Since rigidity develops as a means to block out painful sensations, the release of rigidity or the restoration of the natural motility of the body will bring these painful sensations to the fore. Somewhere in his unconscious the neurotic individual is aware that pleasure can evoke the repressed ghosts of the past. It could be that such a situation is responsible for the adage "No pleasure without pain."

In the human being the primary mechanism for the release of tension is the convulsive discharge of crying. Most infants cry when they are in distress; all infants cry with pain. On the interpersonal or psychological level their crying is a call for the mother. Biologically it is a rebound from a state of contraction. If one observes a baby just before it begins to cry, one will notice how it has stiffened from its distress or pain. Its vibrant and alive body cannot maintain the rigidity. First its jaw begins to quiver, then its chin crumples, and in a moment its whole body is convulsed with its crying. Mothers know that crying is a signal of distress, and hasten to remove the disturbance. The baby, however, does not cry to summon its mother, for it will continue to cry as long as the tension persists.

The function of crying to reduce tension is seen in psychiatric practice. Patients almost invariably declare that they feel better after a good cry. Some patients will even remark, "I need to cry." After crying the patient's body is softer, his breathing easier and deeper, his eyes brighter and his skin color better. One can sense the tension leave the patient's body as the crying progresses. When crying fails to have this effect, it is because the patient is too inhibited to give in fully to the convulsion. A sympathetic touch or an understanding remark may release the inhibition in a patient sufficiently to allow a full discharge to occur.

It is a grave injustice to a child or adult to insist that they stop crying. One can comfort a person who is crying which enables him to relax and makes further crying unnecessary; but to humiliate a crying child is to increase his pain, and augment his rigidity. We stop other people from crying because we cannot stand the sounds and movements of their bodies. It threatens our own rigidity. It induces similar feelings in ourselves which we dare not express and it evokes a resonance in our own bodies which we resist.

Crying, that is, sobbing with tears, as far as I know, is a uniquely human form of expression. Other animals may cry out with pain, but their cry is never a sustained convulsive reaction. Crying is an expression of helplessness. It is probably elated to the complete helplessness of the human infant who is unable to relieve his distress or withdraw from a painful situation. Nature has provided this helpless organism with a means of reducing the destructive tensions that arise from situations with which it cannot cope. As the infant grows and gains mobility through increasing coordination, it develops other responses to pain and distress. It can flee in fear or attack in anger, but these emotions are unavailable to the very young infant.

LECTURE II: THE SPECTRUM OF EMOTIONS

A Hierarchy of Functions

Consciousness arises from an organism's awareness of the sensations produced by the body's activities. Since these sensations are perceived as feeling tones, "every span of consciousness has the quality of either pleasure or pain."[2] Conscious regulation of behavior, that is, the striving for pleasure and to avoid pain, rests upon this basic awareness of body sensation. The absence of sensation, motor or sensory, leads to a disintegration of consciousness.

With the growth and development of consciousness in the human organism, these pleasure-pain sensations become elaborated into emotions. The word, e-motion, describes a movement "out, out of or from," according to the meaning attached to the prefix. An emotion, then, is a movement that arises out of or from an excited state of pleasure or pain. Sandor Rado divides emotions into two groups: the welfare emotions and the emergency emotions. The welfare emotions, which include affection, sympathy and love, are "differentiated elaborations of the experiencing and anticipation of pleasure." The emergency emotions, which induce fear, anger and hate, are "differentiated elaborations of the experiencing and expectation of pain."[3]

Emotions may also be classified according to whether they are simple or compound. A simple emotion leads to a direct action. In anger one attempts to strike out, in fear to get away. Two or more emotions may combine, however, to produce a more complicated response. In resentment, for example, there is anger plus fear covered with a layer of hostility. When emotions are mixed with value judgments the result is a conceptual emotion or feeling. Guilt, shame and vanity fall into this category of emotions.

On the next level of development, feelings and emotions become differentiated into thought. This involves the translation of feelings into symbols and the closer association of feelings with events in the external world. One cannot think of anger without attempting to relate it to a cause. Thinking introduces the question, "Why?" The more one thinks the more one attempts to understand causal relationships. In thinking, the emphasis shifts from the feeling to the stimulus which provoked the feeling, from the action which would follow the feeling or emotion to an understanding and appreciation of the relationship between the stimulus and the feeling.

In emotional thought, the role of the feeling in evoking the thought is explicitly or implicitly recognized and accepted. It is explicit when I think, I am angry because you did something that caused me pain. It is implicit in the thought, What a beautiful day. In the latter case, I implicitly associate the state of the weather with my feeling of pleasure.

A higher level of consciousness enables me to think without reference to feelings. Unemotional thought or logic purportedly deals only with symbols: words, mathematical signs, abstract forces, etc. The connection of the thought content with emotions or feelings is explicitly denied. The thought process is supposed to follow abstract laws which are free of emotional contamination. Such objective thinking is called reasoning to denote the use of a special faculty, the intellect. Reasoning strives for objectivity as opposed to emotional thought which has a strong subjective basis. Human beings have this special faculty of observing and criticizing their own thought processes. This is possible because the human ego is capable of viewing the body somewhat as an object, that is, with detachment; but to believe that the ego is ever fully independent of bodily processes is an illusion. Psychoanalysis has shown that what we think and why we think it are determined by unconscious forces. The distinction, therefore, between subjective and objective, between emotional thought and reason is a difference of degree. Each step in the progression from sensation to emotion and finally to thought represents a higher degree of consciousness. Objective thought or reason is an expression of the highest level of consciousness, the consciousness of the self or the ego.

The whole structure of consciousness with its mechanisms for regulating behavior is rooted in unconscious bodily processes which maintain the life functions of the organism. These processes, hormonal, cellular, chemical and energetic, constitute what Walter Cannon called the wisdom of the body. The relationship of the different levels to each other can be shown diagrammatically as shown in Figure 1 below. In this lecture I shall discuss some of the different emotional responses.

The Simple Emotions

The development of human consciousness is related to the growth and coordination of the muscular system. Before the end of the first year of life a child begins to react to pain and distress by active movements. Quite early he will manifest feelings of irritation which he expresses by random kicking movements. As he grows stronger his irritation will change to anger. From merely pushing away a distasteful object, he will strike out with his arms when frustrated or in pain. This reaction of anger slowly supersedes crying as a means of releasing tension. In the young child, however, anger is generally impotent to change his situation and it usually subsides in to crying which is the more primordial tension-releasing mechanism.

Adult patients in therapy, mostly women, show a similar regression to crying when their attempts at anger prove impotent. Women find it easier to cry than men, who because of their greater muscular development react more quickly with anger to pain. Crying is a more involuntary response to anger and less subject, therefore, to ego control. Anger requires an ability to discriminate a cause for the pain; it implies an object against which the anger is directed. Generally anger is a more effective response than crying since it aims to remove the cause of the pain. Whereas crying gives one a feeling of helplessness in a situation, anger overcomes the feeling of being helpless.

In anger, the excitation charges the muscular system releasing powerful movements of the upper part of the body. The aggressive organs are located in the upper and front end of the body probably because aggression is intimately connected with the seizure of food. People experience anger as an upward surge of feeling charging into the head and arms. When inhibitions exist that block the discharge of this feeling, a tension headache may result. Crying, on the other hand, is experienced as a letting down. The feeling flows downward and the charge recedes from the musculature. Anger is like a storm in many respects. After the feeling is discharged, the brow clears and good feelings return.

Anger belongs to the group of emergency emotions. It activates the sympathetic adrenal system and is a reaction to a feeling of pain. All emotions which belong to this group have the same direction; the feeling surges toward the front and upper end of the body. The emotions which arise from pleasure, the welfare emotions as designated by Rado, have an opposite direction, toward the lower end of the body.

Each emotion can be manifested in a variety of forms which constitute a spectrum of that emotion. The spectrum for anger is shown below. In its mildest form anger appears as annoyance, in its most severe form as fury.

Annoyance•Irritation•Anger•Rage•Fury

Annoyance is felt when the distress is slight. We attempt to rid ourselves of an annoying object with easy movements such as brushing away a fly.

Irritation means that the excitation is building up in the muscular system but that it has not reached the point where it explodes in aggressive action. Irritation results in stronger movements than annoyance.

Anger is a response to pain. Anger denotes that the excitation in the muscular system has reached a boiling point. The release, though involuntary, is subject to ego control which adjusts the action to the reality of the situation. Anger is not destructive.

Rage is a reaction to severe pain such as torment. The muscular excitation is excessive and ego participation in the expression of the feeling is diminished. In contrast to anger, rage has a destructive quality.

Fury is like a whirlwind in that discrimination is absent and ego control is lost.

Fear, like anger, is a reaction to pain or the threat of it. The threat of pain is experienced as painful and our reaction to the threat is the same as to pain. Fear, like anger, is an emergency emotion which activates the sympathetic-adrenal system and mobilizes the musculature of the body. In anger, however, the organism attacks the source of pain, in fear it withdraws and flees from it. In anger the excitation moves forward over the top of the head and into the canines. In fear the excitation withdraws into the back of the neck, pulling the head backward and raising the shoulders. The correspondence between the two emotions is such that if the direction of movement is reversed, one changes into the other. If a frightened person turns to attack, he will become angry and unafraid. When an attacking person starts to retreat, he will feel fear. The spectrum of fear shows the correspondence between the two states of excitation.

Apprehension•Anxiety•Fear•Panic•Terror

Apprehension arises when a situation that promises pleasure also contains the possibility of pain. One is apprehensive that the anticipated pleasure will be lost (pain) but one still moves forward.

Anxiety develops when the threat of pain is approximately equal to the promise of pleasure. In consequence, the organism is caught between two conflicting impulses, to move forward and to withdraw. Anxiety has been reproduced experimentally in animals by coupling a painful stimulus with a pleasurable one. If this is done often enough, the animal associates pain with the pleasurable stimulus and reacts with anxiety to the sight of the latter. In the conflict between the two impulses it is unable to move and shakes violently as the excitation flows through its body.

Fear occurs when pain or the threat of pain dominates the situation producing a desire to escape or withdraw. In animals the attack of anger is generally reserved for the circumstance where withdrawal is physically or psychologically destructive. This concept is explored in Robert Ardrey's book, "The Territorial Imperative." An animal will attack its own species in defense of its status or its territory. I mention this because the question may arise what determines whether the reaction to pain will be fear or anger? If the pain or the threat is overwhelming, one flees in panic or is rooted in terror. Otherwise it could be said, speaking generally, that anger will predominate if one is convinced that he is right.

Panic is an overriding fear. One's only impulse is to get away, and the impulse is so strong that one runs blindly. It is related to claustrophobia, a feeling of being trapped or of the walls closing in on one. In panic a person finds his breath cut off. Fright normally causes a person to suck in air. This is an emergency mechanism to provide extra oxygen for flight. When the fear increases to panic, the air is held, the throat closes and the chest becomes rigid. It is locked in the inspiratory position. The person cannot breathe and this increases his panic. The moment the person escapes the danger his breathing returns to normal.

Terror is a more severe form of fright than panic. In terror the musculature is paralyzed making fight or flight impossible. Terror develops in situations of overwhelming pain or danger. Feeling is withdrawn from the periphery of the body to reduce the organism's sensitivity to the final agony. It is a literal flight inward. Terror is equivalent to a state of shock. The loss of muscle tone in terror causes the breath to be expelled and makes inspiration almost impossible. The chest is held in an expiratory position. Terror may cause a person to faint, in which case life is maintained by the unconscious bodily processes. If terror is prolonged, it leads to a depersonalization, that is, a dissociation of the perceiving ego from the body.

The developing consciousness of the child enables it to recognize the specific sources of its pleasure, to recall past satisfaction and

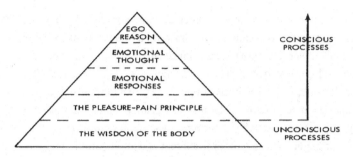

Fig. 1 The Simple Emotions

anticipate future joys. The anticipation of pleasure evokes a positive feeling for the object that is the source of the pleasure. This feeling may be described in its simplest form as affection. Whereas anger and fear have their roots in painful sensations, affection arises from pleasurable sensations. Rado would describe it as a welfare emotion. It activates the parasympathetic system which expands the body and produces feelings that flow downward. The downward feeling may be explained as establishing contact with the ground or earth, which is a symbol for the mother from whom all affection flows.

Affection varies in depth depending on the intensity of the anticipated pleasure. The following is a suggested spectrum of this feeling.

Friendliness•Amity•Affection•Fondness•Love

Friendliness differentiates our feelings for those who share similar tastes and attitudes from the feelings we have for a stranger. Pleasures are shared with friends.

Amity is very similar to friendship. It includes the idea of good will towards others.

Affection is a feeling of warmth towards someone. The warmth is a real physical sensation produced by the dilation of the peripheral blood vessels under the action of the parasympathetic nervous system. This feeling is more personal than the preceding two.

Fondness may be denoted as a special feeling for a person that is more defined than affection but less intense than love.

Love implies the strongest desire for closeness with another and promises the greatest pleasure. In our minds ecstasy is associated with sexuality, the most intimate relationship of two people, but such a high degree of pleasure is possible only when sex is an expression of love. This seems to be very rare in our culture.

Affectionate feelings are rooted in the experience of pleasure and linked to the anticipation of pleasure. A person who is limited in his ability to feel pleasure is limited in his capacity to love. A person who is afraid of pleasure is afraid to love. The ability to love grows out of a child's experience of pleasure in its relation to its parents, especially its mother. This intimate connection between pleasure and love shows the importance of pleasure in life. Without pleasure, a person is blocked from the experiences which give life its true meaning. With little pleasure, one can survive in a detached and unrelated existence while clinging to the illusion that someday he will find the love that will transfuse his life with joy. Unfortunately this doesn't happen; pleasure is an essential ingredient of love. The inevitable collapse of the illusion leaves the person bitter and disenchanted.

Affection or love is an expansive reaction, a reaching out to others and the world. Affectionate people are pleasure-loving, outgoing, warm, relaxed and sweet. They are sweet because pleasure is sweet. In the absence of pleasure a person turns bitter. The bitter person is cold, withdrawn and tense. Love turns cold when the pleasure goes out of a relationship.

When the relation of a child to its parents is charged with painful experiences, the child develops feelings of hostility which are often covered over with pious protestations of love. The association of a person or situation with painful sensations gives rise to the hostile emotions. These form a spectrum that ranges from unfriendly feelings to hate. There is a correspondence between the hostile emotion and the affectionate ones.

It is not difficult to understand the polarity of love and hate. In my first book, I defined hate as frozen love, that is, as love turned ice cold. Since every relationship is based on an expectation of pleasure, its outcome can only be fulfillment or disappointment. The degree of disappointment will be proportionate to the expectation of pleasure if that pleasure is not realized. Disappointment is a painful sensation. It undermines the harmony between our inner feeling of rhythm and the environment. The rejection of affection in a relationship is experienced as a deep hurt which produces feelings of hostility.

The following spectrum suggests a range of hostile feelings.

Unfriendliness•Enmity•Hostility•Antipathy•Hate

Unfriendliness is the attitude one has towards a stranger who does not pose a threat. Many years ago I saw a cartoon in which two Welshmen were standing together watching a stranger approach. "D'ye know 'im, Bill?" asks the first. "No," answers the second Welshman. "'Eve a rock at 'im," says the first one.

I believe we are naturally unfriendly to strangers. In modern civilization hospitality to the stranger is a concept that has to be taught either as part of the Judao-Christian tradition or some other. Among children the newcomer is viewed with reserve. He, in turn, approaches an established group of children cautiously. He watches their activities from the periphery for some time and very gradually moves closer. In time his familiarity insures his acceptance.

The stranger represents a disturbing element in the feeling of ease and harmony which pervades a group. His presence inhibits the flow of pleasurable sensations that takes place between intimates and evokes, therefore, some degree of hostility. The more different he is, the greater the disturbance his presence causes and the stronger the negative reactions to him. On the other hand, the stranger introduces novelty and excitement with their promise of pleasure. Which of the two factors will determine the response to a stranger depends on the personality of the group members. A secure individual will accept a stranger more readily than an insecure one, but this acceptance follows an initial caution or coldness.

The persecution of the stranger is an expression of hate rather than simple unfriendliness. Since he is a natural object for hostile feelings, he easily becomes a target for the repressed hatreds that stem from painful childhood experiences. People project on the stranger the intense hostilities that were evoked in the home and repressed through the operation of guilt. The stranger becomes the scapegoat to whom these hostilities are transferred. Such a transference generally meets with social approval and is often rationalized by the ego. The unfriendliness that frequently greets the stranger is gradually overcome by increasing familiarity but the hatred of the stranger cannot be resolved socially.

Repressed hatreds require a therapeutic situation for their release. First, some form of analytic technique must be used to make these hatreds conscious. Second, the guilt which serves to keep these hostile feelings suppressed must be worked through. And third, some means must be provided for the expression of the hostility in the controlled setting of the therapeutic situation so that the physical tensions which underlie the negative feelings are released. Hostilities are abreacted, that is, vented and discharged, when they are expressed in appropriate forms of anger. When this occurs, the capacity of the individual to experience pleasure is restored and "good feelings" become the normal tone of the body.

Enmity is a more intense feeling than unfriendliness. It is reserved for strangers who are considered a threat.

Hostility is the generic term for this class of emotions. Broadly speaking, hostility is manifested in coldness and withdrawal. If a person is cold to another he is said to be hostile. Hostility does not denote an aggressive action. It refers to an attitude. A hostile action combines a negative attitude with some form of anger.

Antipathy may be viewed as the opposite of fondness. It denotes such an intense dislike that one avoids contact with another.

Hate has been explained above as the opposite of love. The expression of hatred in action is either rage or fury. Unexpressed, it is manifested in a rigidity of the body, that is, in a freezing of all spontaneous motility.

It can be said that we are hostile to people of whom we are afraid, but it is equally true that we are afraid of people towards whom we feel hostile. This is because both emotions have the anticipation of pain as a common element. When we're hostile, we are on guard, prepared to attack but also to flee if that becomes necessary. Lowering one's guard is a sign of affection, an indication that one anticipates pleasure from a meeting rather than pain.

The maturation of the organism with its expanding consciousness also introduces the memories of past pleasures and pains as significant emotions. The recall of a past pleasure is a present pleasure. We look back to our pleasurable experiences with affection. However, the recall of past pain has special qualities. If the pain was caused by the loss of a love object or a source of pleasure, the recollection gives rise to the emotion of sadness. This emotion is evoked by the memory of the pleasure which has been lost; the pain of the loss is only indirectly perceived. Sadness is, therefore, considered by Rado to be a welfare emotion which is mediated by the parasympathetic system and has an underlying tone of pleasure. It elicits a positive response from people.

Sadness normally leads to crying but this reaction is different from the child's crying as a result of pain. All crying releases tension which cannot be released any other way. The child cries because it is helpless to remove a present source of pain. An adult cries because he is also helpless to restore a lost love object. In the first case anger is unavailable, in the second case, it is meaningless.

Reflecting its origin, sadness has a bitter-sweet quality. This quality determines a spectrum for this emotion.

Sadness•Sorrow•Grief

Sadness occurs when the memory of the good feelings outweighs the pain.

Sorrow is a feeling in which the pain of the loss outweighs the memory of the pleasure.

Grief develops when the pain dominates the picture to the exclusion of the pleasure. Grief is a bitter emotion.

Patients in therapy will often feel sad and cry without being aware of the reason for their feeling. They often remark, "I do not know why I feel sad." The immediate occasion for the sadness is the recapture of sensation in parts of the body that were blocked from consciousness. In effect, a person's body is his original love object, the real source of pleasure. Making contact with a forsaken body[4] activates the sense of loss and arouses the feeling of sadness. As the feeling of sadness grows stronger, it will embrace the loss of contact with the mother's body, the first environmental source of pleasure, and later it will be extended to include the loss of love between the parents and the child.

The Repression of Emotion - Illusion

Closely related to the emotion of sadness is the loss of feeling known as depression. The term describes what happens, a depression of all vital functions and a corresponding loss of feeling and motivation. On the other hand, depression is a feeling since we do sense our lowered responsiveness.

When the threat of losing a love object produces a pain so severe that it imperils the integrity of the organism, the impending catastrophe is denied by the consciousness and replaced by an illusion. The illusion serves to sustain the spirit against what appears to the person as an irreparable loss. Illusion is the antidote to despair, the corollary of desperation. Its role is discussed in *The Betrayal of the Body*. Two examples will illustrate its connection with depression.

The Voice of the Body

A child in despair about its parents' love may develop an illusion that if he becomes famous, the world, a symbol for the parents, will adore him and love him. Throughout his life this child will desperately try to fulfill this dream, unaware that he is laboring under an illusion, since fame never brought true love. In similar circumstances another child may develop the illusion that obedience and productivity will insure the return of the lost love. In both cases, the sacrifice of pleasure which the illusion demands makes success a meaningless victory. Sooner or later, the bubble will burst, the dream will fade and the illusion will collapse. Their energies exhausted in a desperate maneuver to fulfill an impossible image, both persons will become depressed. Unaware of the illusion to which they have subordinated all feeling, they cannot understand the reason for their depression.

I introduced the concept of depression here because of its direct connection with sadness and the other emotions. The depressed person is neither sad nor angry, neither frightened nor hostile. He is, specifically, depressed, which means that his bodily processes are depressed. His appetite is diminished, his motility is reduced and his breathing is restricted. The immediate consequences of this decrease in vital functioning are a lowered energy metabolism and a loss of feeling tone in the body. Depression can be treated psychologically by releasing the repressed emotions. It can be treated physically by activating the bodily functions. A combined approach is most effective.

When the breathing of depressed patients is stimulated through appropriate exercises, they begin to cry. Surprisingly, many of these patients see no reason for their crying. They do not feel sad. They may even ask me, "Why am I crying?" This loss of feeling is the basis of their depression. As the breathing becomes more abdominal through continued physical therapy, the crying deepens into a rhythmic sobbing which restores the motility of the body and lifts the depression. Gradually, patients sense their underlying sadness and gain insight into the loss that provoked it. A sad person is not depressed for where depression leaves an individual cold and unresponsive, a sad person is warm and alive.

The acceptance of sadness opens the door to the experience of pleasure. The reactivation of the pleasure-pain feelings allows the patient to react emotionally with fear and anger to the traumas that inflicted the pain and caused his problem. With the restoration of emotional responsiveness the need for illusions and the tendency to depression are overcome.

The Mixed Emotions

Human beings can discriminate many feelings which are mixtures of the simple emotions described above. Compassion, for example, combines both affection and sadness. *Webster's International Dictionary* defines the root of this word as "to bear or suffer with another." Without a feeling of affection which unites one person to another, the suffering of others would leave us cold. We identify with persons towards whom we feel affectionate and we can share their sorrow because we have known our own. Compassion means "with feeling for another." It includes sympathy and pity. Our sympathy extends to another person in distress, our pity is a response to his pain.

Closely allied to the feeling of sympathy is the phenomenon of empathy which enables us to sense what other people are feeling. The empathic understanding takes place on the body level. We are sensitive to the rhythmic movements in other people's bodies if our own bodies are alive and responsive, that is, if our own rhythmic activity is free and undisturbed. The alive body vibrates like a tuning fork. It has the capacity, therefore, to resonate in harmony with other bodies. What we perceive through empathy is the resonance in our body as it responds to the vibration in others. A rigid person lacks this capacity.

People who share a sense of community are affected by one another. Within a community feelings are contagious. We become sad in the presence of a sad person and feel uplifted in the presence of a joyful person. Like sympathy, the empathic understanding only extends, however, to those towards whom we feel some affection. Painful feelings and the emotions which derive from them, fear, anger and hostility, block the empathic understanding. And when feelings are suppressed by chronic tensions, the sense of empathy diminishes.

Pleasure is the key to the empathic response. Without good feelings in our own body, we lack the ability to reach out to others on the preverbal level at which empathy occurs. Pleasure is, therefore, the base for all meaningful interpersonal relationships. When pleasure is ignored or its importance denied, relationships disintegrate into conflict. This is especially true in the home, where closeness and intimacy encourage a great expectation of pleasure. A home without joy is a scene of discord in which no one seems to be able to understand or sympathize with the difficulties and sufferings of the others.

Another compound emotion is resentment which is composed of hostility and fear. The fear prevents the hostility from being openly expressed as anger with the result that resentment is a smoldering emotion. The resentful person harbors his hostility until it swells and becomes greater than his fear at which time it explodes as rage. If the fear is too great to allow any release, the resentment turns into spite. The hostility turns inward and is expressed in self-destructive actions which have the unconscious purpose of destroying the other person's good feeling. One can only be spiteful against someone who cares.

Envy, another compound emotion, is a combination of sadness plus hostility. The envious person has suffered a loss of pleasure. This makes him sad but he cannot release the sadness because of guilt. His guilt makes him hostile but he cannot express his hostility either. The hostility becomes directed against the person who has not suffered a loss of pleasure. Unable to share a feeling of joy, the envious person wants to deprive the other person of his good fortune. I believe we all sense the hostility behind envy. Included in the spectrum of envy are the emotions of bitterness and jealousy. In jealousy, the hostility leads to overt action; the jealous person cannot tolerate the other person's pleasure. The bitter person, on the other hand, turns the hostility against himself and withdraws inward to nurture his pain.

One more compound emotion will suffice to illustrate this concept. Awe combines both pleasure and fear. An awesome spectacle is exciting and fearful; its exciting aspect entices the observer to approach while its fearful aspect makes him want to run away. The effect of these two opposite feelings acting together is to leave the observer suspended in a state of awe.

Where antithetical emotions occur at the same time, we speak of mixed feelings or ambivalence. Thus, love and hate can coexist in a person with regard to the same object. We may be attracted by some features of an object and repelled by others. We can be both frightened and angry at the same time, or simultaneously want to laugh and to cry. Whether ambivalent or mixed feelings are normal or neurotic can only be understood with reference to a specific situation. Their consequence in all cases is to block any effective response to the situation since they do not fuse into a definite reaction.

When an individual is suspended between two conflicting impulses he is forced to use the power of thought to resolve the impasse. One of the two conflicting impulses is suppressed in favor of the other. If the suppression of a feeling is coupled with a moral judgment, the result is what I call a "conceptual emotion." Mixed feelings are generally resolved by practical judgments, the normal solution to this problem.

The Conceptual Emotions

A feeling of guilt is a conceptual emotion. It represents the imposition of a moral judgment upon a bodily function or process, which is beyond the control of the ego or conscious mind. To understand this idea, a distinction should be drawn between guilt as a legal judgment and guilt as a moral judgment. The former is a determination of action or behavior which contravenes an established law. The latter gives rise to a feeling which often bears no relation to one's actions or behavior. A person who breaks a law is guilty of a crime whether he feels guilty or not. A child who has hostility against his parents can feel guilty though he has committed no destructive act. The feeling of guilt is not a judgment of behavior but a judgment placed upon emotions.

Sexual desires are a common source of guilt feelings. But a sexual desire is a natural body response to a state of excitation which is normally beyond the control of the ego or mind. It has its origin in the pleasure functions of the body. To feel guilty about sexual desire is to turn against the body. To suppress a sexual desire is to depress all pleasure functions of the body. On the other hand, to accept one's sexual feelings does not mean that one has the right to act upon them in any situation. A healthy ego or personality has the power to control behavior so that it is appropriate to the situation. The lack of this power in a weak ego or a sick personality may lead to actions which are destructive to individuals and destructive to the social order. Society has the right and obligation to protect its members against such behavior. It has no right to label the feeling itself as wrong.

A feeling of guilt denotes that a part of the personality, the ego, has turned against another part, the feelings of the body. This split in the unity of the personality produces destructive effects which are explored in *The Betrayal of the Body*. The major part of all psychotherapeutic effort is directed at removing the feeling of guilt in order to restore the integrity of the personality. It is precisely the feeling of guilt that undermines the ego's power to control behavior. This is not to say that a healthy person is perfect. We can all do things that hurt others, and when we do, our reaction should be regret or sorrow, true emotions.

Every feeling or emotion can become an object of guilt if a moral judgment is attached to it. Generally, it is our sexual or hostile feelings which become colored by such judgments. Unfortunately, most people are unaware of their guilt feelings since these are repressed together with the forbidden desire. This overall suppression reduces the pleasure of living. By denying themselves pleasure, people avoid their anxiety and hide their guilt.

Just as some feelings are judged morally wrong, others are judged to be morally superior. The person who feels righteous has suppressed his hostility in favor of a pseudo-affection, his anger in favor of a facade of compassion, and his pleasure in favor of his ego image. He has also repressed his guilt about his true feelings. Righteousness and guilt are like the head and tail of a coin. One does not exist without the other, although only one shows at a time. Every person who feels guilt carries a hidden feeling of moral superiority.

Another conceptual emotion is the feeling of shame. This feeling denotes a negative judgment placed upon the body and its biological processes. To the ego the body is a corrupt thing, fated to deteriorate and decay whereas the mind, pure and incorporeal, is infinite and immortal. The shame of the body causes us to reject it and dissociate from it. Like the feeling of guilt, it splits the unity of the personality. It makes us overly self-conscious of our appearance. It leads necessarily to feelings of vanity and conceit. Vanity implies a positive judgment of the body, clothed or naked, which covers an underlying feeling of shame. The conceited person is preoccupied with his image and rejects his body. The normal feelings about the body which are free from value judgments are modesty and pride. In his modesty and pride, a person expresses his identification with his body and his pleasure and joy in its functioning.

The spectrum of emotions analyzed above is necessarily incomplete. I have omitted such feelings as remorse whose components are obscure. Feelings and emotions are subject to gradations which words are not fully capable of describing. In this lecture I have attempted to show the relation of emotions to the feelings of pleasure and pain which underlie them. Superimposed upon the emotions are the processes of the mind. The connection between feeling and thinking will be the subject of a future discussion.

LECTURE III: THE RHYTHMIC MOVEMENTS OF THE BODY

Rhythms of Natural Functions

In the first lecture pleasure was defined as the conscious perception of the rhythmic and pulsatory activity of the body produced by an inner state of excitation. Any disturbance of this rhythmic activity will produce some sensation of pain. The intensity of the pleasure or pain is proportionate to the degree of excitation.

The growth of consciousness and the ego plus the development of motor coordination lead to the elaboration and differentiation of emotions from the broad feelings of pleasure and pain. Emotions are organized states of excitation related to specific situations in the environment. A further differentiation occurs with the development of speech which permits the abstraction of feeling-states from direct motor action and their expression in words. Increasing abstraction through the use of words as symbols results in the higher forms of thinking such as logic. Man has been so fascinated by his ability to manipulate symbols and gain knowledge that he has tended to overlook the fact that the base of this structure consists of the involuntary processes of his body. In this study I will point out some of the body's rhythmic activities and show their relation to the experience of pleasure and pain.

The most obvious bodily rhythm is the alternance between sleep and wakefulness. For most animals, including man, this alternance corresponds roughly to the diurnal rhythm of day and night. During the day we are conscious and active, at night consciousness is surrendered and activity is reduced. It can be said that in sleep the body renews itself; it has been shown that any prolonged deprivation of sleep produces severe disturbances in the body and the personality. The phenomenon of sleep, however, is still as mysterious as that of pleasure. I like to think that in sleep we return to a vegetative type of existence similar in some respects to plant life, a mode of existence from which the animal departed at the start of its evolution. But this is pure speculation.

Sleep is a state of diffused and lowered excitation. In sleep many vital functions of the body show a reduced rhythmicity: the heart beats more slowly, blood pressure drops, there is a decrease in blood sugar, the respiratory rate diminishes, and the body temperature lowers. Electroencephalograms show that there are cycles during sleep, a rhythmic rise and fall in the level of excitation which changes the depth of sleep. If the process of sleep is undisturbed, a person awakens with a feeling of having been refreshed, an eagerness to start the day's activities and, normally, a desire for food. Rising from a good night's sleep, one feels a distinct sensation of pleasure, as if the body were somehow aware during sleep of its harmonious functioning. Similarly, going to sleep when one is tired but relaxed is a most delightful sensation.

This simple pleasure escapes many people, if we can judge by the demand for sleep-inducing pills. These people complain of being tired and their need for sleep evident yet they do not fall asleep when they go to bed. Obviously, in such cases something is wrong with the normal self-regulating processes of the body. I discussed some aspects of this situation in *The Betrayal of the Body*. The inability to fall asleep is a form of falling anxiety, an anxiety about the loss of consciousness. On another level, this anxiety reflects the persistence of a state of excitation in the conscious layers of the personality. Sometimes the persistent excitation is an undischarged sexual tension but more often it is due to residual fears and anxieties left over from the day's activities. If the persistent excitation is unconscious, it will manifest itself in dreams which, as Freud pointed out, have the function of guarding the state of slumber by releasing the excitation. However, the excitation may be so strong that the person is awakened by the dream, or the restfulness of his sleep is disturbed by the intensity of the dream.

The bodily functions related to food, ingestion, digestion and elimination follow a rhythmic pattern governed by the energy needs of the organism. Very young infants nurse as often as every two hours and have several bowel movements a day. In adults the pattern tends to become stabilized at three meals and one bowel movement a day. Eating

77

is a pleasure when it conforms to an internal rhythm. Too many people, however, are compulsive eaters; their food habits bear little relation to their metabolic rhythms. They eat before they are hungry, probably to avoid the feeling of hunger since this feeling is associated with sensations of emptiness that are frightening to affection-starved individuals.

Compulsive eaters do not enjoy their food. The initial pleasure of putting something tasty into their mouths is not followed by the deeper satisfaction that comes from assuaging hunger. For them, eating is a sensual pleasure which, like all other sensual pleasures, leaves one unfulfilled. The sensation of being stuffed and overfull, while distinctly unpleasant, temporarily overcomes the feelings of emptiness and anxiety which underlie compulsive eating. Since these gnawing sensations soon reappear, a vicious circle is created that leads to more eating. People are also compulsive about the function of elimination. They develop a habit of regularity based on rigid toilet training which substitutes a spurious ego satisfaction for the pleasure of a spontaneous elimination.

The digestive tract from mouth to anus is a rhythmically pulsating organ system which functions very much like a worm. Food is moved from one end of this tube to the other by peristaltic waves similar to the waves which pass through the body of a worm or a caterpillar as it moves forward. Along the digestive tube there are constrictions and enlargements, such as the stomach, which facilitate the digestive process and modify the frequency and form of the rhythmic wave but do not change its essential character. Since this peristaltic activity is always present, there is a continuing excitation in the digestive tract, higher at meal times, lower during sleep. When this excitation is maintained within normal limits, the person has a "good feeling" in his body. A hyperactive state in any part of the system, a condition of colitis for example, replaces the normal good feeling tone with painful sensations. Hypotonicity or loss of tone in any segment produces feelings of distress.

We are generally unconscious of the normal functioning of the alimentary canal from a point below the pharynx to another above the rectum. The conscious pleasure of eating good food lies in its ability to excite the taste buds, the salivary glands and the reflex of deglutition, that is, the area from the mouth to the esophagus. This excitation, however, passes through the whole alimentary canal quickening its rhythms and stimulating its secretion. Thus, the initial pleasure of taste is transformed into enjoyment of food. When tensions exist in the tube which block the easy flow of the peristaltic waves, we are denied this deeper satisfaction and even the pleasure we anticipate from the taste of food decreases. We may even lose our appetite or feel sick at the stomach.

Few conditions make a person feel as miserable as sensations of nausea. The body seems to revolt at its core and seeks to disgorge itself of the noxious substance. The nausea produces severe peristaltic waves which move upward, increasing in intensity until the body heaves up this offending substance. Vomiting produces a sense of relief which is as great as the preceding distress but the experience is never a pleasurable one.

The mechanism of vomiting is a protective reflex against dangerous or harmful substances which have been swallowed in error. But it can also be evoked by tension states, especially the stress of emotional conflict while one is eating. Almost everyone has had experiences of this kind. I recall an incident when my child was one year old which illustrates this idea. We had just finished lunch and were rushing to leave for an appointment. While my wife was dressing the baby, he suddenly put his finger in his mouth and threw up his meal. I was surprised that a child so young would know how to relieve his distress by gagging himself.

Patients in bioenergetic therapy occasionally develop feelings of nausea in the course of their efforts to breathe more deeply. The nausea seems to be independent of food intake for it may happen to a patient some hours after a light breakfast. It seems that the deeper breathing activates chronic tensions in the diaphragm and stomach which then produce this feeling of nausea. In some cases, the nausea can be relieved by abdominal breathing which relaxes the diaphragm. In other cases, the feeling is intensified by this procedure and the patient has to throw up to release the tension.

In part the origin of this tension lies in childhood feeding experiences; children are often made to eat food which they do not like or in amounts which they do not want. Many jokes have been made about mothers who in the name of love overstuff their children. In other homes, as patients have told me, the children are forbidden to leave the table until they have finished everything on their plates. Not only is a child often made to eat food that conflicts with his desire, but he is shamed and scolded if he should throw it up. To hold it down, the child must tense his diaphragm, blocking off any impulse to vomit.

Food is not the only thing a person may have to swallow against his wishes. Psychological traumas such as insults and humiliations may also have to be "swallowed" when one is afraid of the insulting person. The expression "I can't stomach it" indicates the effect on this organ of submission to painful situations. In addition, children are often forced to "swallow" their tears or their crying which leads to chronic tensions in the throat and diaphragm. Since there is hardly a patient who hasn't suffered such traumas, it is to be expected that a therapy which works directly with the physical tensions of the body would activate the suppressed impulse to "throw it up." However, most patients find it difficult to throw up easily. It often requires considerable work on the gag reflex before the throat and diaphragmatic tensions are sufficiently released to allow this function to operate normally. One result of this procedure is the elimination of chronic heartburn which plagues so many people. In all cases, the release of the diaphragmatic tension restores the pleasure to the basic activities of eating and digestion and facilitates a fuller respiration.

The respiratory system is closely allied to the alimentary canal. Its function is disturbed by the conflicts which stem from the denial of the pleasure principle underlying self-regulation of the digestive system. Embryologically, the lungs develop as an outgrowth of the primitive alimentary tube and throughout life they remain connected to this tube through the mouth and pharynx. We take in air as we take in food. Air is sucked into our bodies just as milk is sucked by an infant from its mother's breast. And, as Margaret Ribble showed in her important book, *The Rights of Infants*, any weakening of the sucking impulse depresses the respiratory function. It is a common belief that we breathe with our lungs alone, but in point of fact, the work of breathing is done by the whole body. The lungs play a passive role in the respiratory process. Their expansion is produced by an enlargement, mostly downward, of the thoracic cavity and they collapse when that cavity is reduced. Proper breathing involves the muscles of the head, neck, thorax, and abdomen. It can be shown that chronic tension in any part of the body's musculature interferes with the natural respiratory movements.

Breathing is a rhythmic activity. Normally a person at rest makes approximately 16 to 17 respiratory incursions a minute. The rate is higher in infants and in states of excitation. It is lower in sleep and in depressed persons. The depth of the respiratory wave is another factor which varies with emotional states. Breathing becomes shallow when we are frightened or anxious. It deepens with relaxation, pleasure and sleep. But above all, it is the quality of the respiratory movements that determines whether breathing is pleasurable or not. With each breath a wave can be seen to ascend and descend through the body. The inspiratory wave begins deep in the abdomen with a backward movement of the pelvis. This allows the belly to expand outward. The wave then moves upward as the rest of the body expands. The head moves very slightly forward to suck in the air while the nostrils dilate or the mouth opens. The expiratory wave begins in the upper part of the body and moves downward: the head drops back, the chest and abdomen collapse, and the pelvis rocks forward.

Breathing easily and fully is one of the basic pleasures of being alive. The pleasure is clearly experienced at the end of expiration when the descending wave fills the pelvis with a delicious sensation. In adults this sensation has a sexual quality, though it does not induce any genital feeling. The slight backward and forward movements of the pelvis, similar to the sexual movements, add to the pleasure. Though the rhythm of breathing is pronounced in the pelvic area, it is at the same time experienced by the total body as a feeling of fluidity, softness, lightness and excitement.

The importance of breathing need hardly be stressed. It provides the oxygen for the metabolic processes; literally it supports the fires of life. But breath as "pneuma" is also the spirit or soul. We live in an ocean of air like fish in a body of water. By our breathing we are attuned to our atmosphere. If we inhibit our breathing we isolate ourselves from the medium in which we exist. In all Oriental and mystic philosophies, the breath holds the secret to the highest bliss. That is why breathing is the dominant factor in the practice of Yoga.

Rhythms of Movement

The rhythmic activities of the body can be divided into three categories: those related to the function of the inner tube, digestion and respiration; those related to the outer tube, sensory perception and voluntary movements; and the activities of the organs and structures between them. This division parallels very roughly the embryonic development of the body from the three primary layers: the endoderm, the ectoderm, and the mesoderm. The endoderm gives rise to the skin and nervous system. The latter invaginates and becomes an interior system. From the mesoderm develop the skeleton, heart, blood vessels, glands, musculature and the connective tissues. The voluntary musculature forms a sheath about the body close to the skin and becomes a part of the outer tube. Thus, the body is constructed on the principle of a tube within a tube like a worm.

This division of activities does not imply an independence of one category from the others. The functions of the inner tube, digestion and respiration, are intimately connected with the movements of the outer tube. And both tubes are dependent, or course, on the activities of the organ and tissues which maintain the integrity of the organism.

The outer tube which consists of the skin, the subjacent tissues and striated musculature is directly concerned with the perception of and response to environmental stimuli. For these functions, sensory and motor, it is richly supplied with nerve endings. We are, therefore, more conscious of sensations, especially of sensations of pleasure and pain, in this part of our body than in any other.

Every stimulus that impinges upon the body surface and is perceived by the organism is either pleasurable or painful. Logically, there are no indifferent stimuli, for a stimulus that fails to evoke some sensation would not be perceived. What quality in the stimulus, we may ask, determines whether our response will be pleasurable or painful? Why, for example, are certain sounds delightful to the ear while others are cacophonous and even painful? A cursory knowledge of human beings tells us that such questions cannot be answered objectively. People react differently. What is one man's pleasure is another's pain. So much depends on the mood and manner of the individual receiving the sense impression. There is a big difference between a caress and a slap yet not everyone finds a caress pleasurable nor a slap painful. Children object to being caressed when they are active and a slap on the back may be an expression of appreciation.

Broadly speaking, we find sensory pleasure in stimuli which harmonize with the rhythm and tone of our bodies. Dance music is enjoyable when we wish to dance, disturbing when we are trying to think. Even a favorite symphony can be distracting when one is engaged in a serious conversation. The same thing is true of all the senses. A well prepared meal is a delight to a hungry person, not to one who has no appetite. A charming country scene is pleasurable to behold when we are quiet and contented, not if we are restless and inpatient. Pleasurable sensory impressions not only heighten our mood. they also increase the rhythmic activity of our bodies. They are, simply said, exciting.

Sensory pleasure, it would appear, can be had by everyone in one form or another. But consider the person who is "out of sorts" and finds no pleasure in the sights and sounds about him. Nothing seems to please him. He is, as we say, at sixes and sevens with himself. He is out of sorts because he has no internal harmony. Lacking a consistent tone or pattern of rhythmic activity, he is unable to respond openly and expansively to any environment. The depressed or withdrawn person is in a similar situation. Sensory pleasure or sensual pleasure is unavailable to him because he cannot reach out to the stimulus. But what is depressed in a withdrawn person is his rhythmic activity. Without rhythm there is no pleasure.

The relation of rhythm to pleasure is most clearly seen in the motor function of the outer tube, that is, in the voluntary movements of the body. Any motor activity that is performed rhythmically is pleasurable. Without rhythm the same activity would have a painful quality. The best example is walking. When one walks rhythmically, the walk is enjoyable; when one walks to get to a destination as quickly as possible; the physical activity becomes a chore. Even such a tedious activity as sweeping a floor can be pleasurable when the movements are rhythmical. One can gauge the lack of pleasure in people's lives by the way they move. The rapid, jerky and compulsive movements of most people in our culture betray their lack of joy in life. The person who knows pleasure moves rhythmically, effortlessly and gracefully.

Dancing is, of course, the classic example of pleasure in rhythmic movement. The music sets the beat going in our bodies which is then translated into the rhythmic pattern of the dance step. How painful to feel one's self out of step with the music and how disturbing to find that the music is out of tune with our internal beat. Marching does the same thing for walking that dance music does for dancing. The music accentuates the natural beat in our bodies and by focusing our attention on the rhythm increases our pleasure.

It is important to realize that the music does not create the rhythm. In fact, music is the expression of the rhythm in the composer's body which finds an echo in the body of the listener. It would be correct to say that music evokes the rhythms that are within us. All bodily activity is inherently rhythmical, the movements of the outer tube are no exception. It is simply a matter of coordination. The infant whose sucking movements are coordinated at birth performs this activity rhythmically and pleasurably. Later as he gains increasing coordination over his other movements, these, too, become rhythmical and a source of pleasure to him. Watch a young child jumping on a bed or an older girl jumping rope and you will gain an idea of the pleasure these simple rhythmic activities afford the young.

Adults with their greater coordination require more complex rhythms to feel pleasure. For example, they engage in various sports. No matter what sport a person prefers, it is the rhythmic quality of his movements in that sport that provides his pleasure. I can think of skiing and swimming, two sports I like, as good examples. In both these sports a high degree of coordination is required. When that is achieved and the skiing or swimming takes on a rhythmic quality, the pleasure is great. The moment the rhythm is lost, the activity becomes a painful struggle.

One reason why sports play such a big role in our lives is because our daily activities have lost their rhythmic quality. People walk mechanically, they work compulsively and even talk monotonously, without rhythm and sometimes without rhyme or reason. It may be that the lack of rhythm is due to the lack of pleasure in these activities. It is equally true that the lack of pleasure is due to the loss of rhythm.

We have divided our world into the things we do seriously, for a purpose or gain, and the things we do for fun or pleasure. In the serious affairs of life spontaneous rhythm has no place. We seek the so-called cool efficiency of the machine. We then try hopefully to recover our rhythm and warmth in sports, games and other forms of recreation. But here again we are too often frustrated by our compulsive drive for perfection.

Man is fascinated by the productive efficiency of the machine which can perform any single operation better than he can. The machine gains its efficiency by following one rhythmic pattern. In contrast, man has many rhythmic patterns to correspond to his different moods and desires. He is capable of changing rhythm as his excitement varies. He is capable of weaving complex rhythmic patterns to increase his pleasure and joy. He is, in other words, biologically structured for pleasure not achievement. Man is a creative being not a productive one. Yet, out of his pleasure have come great achievements. Unfortunately, out of his achievement he has found little joy because production has become more important than pleasure.

The operation of the vital organs is not generally associated with pleasure. We are for the most part not aware of their rhythmic activity. We become conscious of them only when something goes wrong and painful sensations develop. Let the heart skip a beat or suddenly increase its rhythm and we are immediately alarmed. We are content, therefore, if nothing occurs to disturb our lack of awareness. Yet these organs, especially the heart, play an important role in our experience of pleasure. To feel good our bodies must be in a state of health which means that "good feelings" reflect an optimum functioning of the vital organs. The heart is, however, directly involved in the more excited pleasurable states.

Rhythm of Love

The joy of love and the love of joy are bodily responses to an excitation that reaches and opens the heart. This is most directly experienced in the sexual act. In the climax of total sexual response the heart races with excitement to complete surrender. Persons who are not conscious of this accelerated rhythm miss the peak of pleasure. Others become frightened and hold back their excitement. If no inhibitions exist against the full surrender to pleasure, the sensation of the heart's rhythmic activity is the height of bliss.

This highest bliss, joy, is the subject of Beethoven's Ninth Symphony. It is also known as the Choral Symphony since it ends with a choral rendition of Schiller's poem, "Ode to Joy." The chorus, as in a Greek tragedy, is intended, I believe, to be a substitute for the audience. Beethoven wanted each listener to experience the feeling of joy in nature and in the brotherhood of man. To do this, he had to reach the hearts of his audience with the music, literally not figuratively, and to make each listener perceive the rhythmic beat of his heart as it pulses in common with the hearts of others.

Beethoven accomplished this objective in the first three movements of the symphony. The first movement depicts the appeal of the individual for love and the response of the universe, Be Joyful. It is so powerful that one of my friends said, "It rips and tears open my chest wall, exposing my heart." The second movement is punctuated from time to time by two loud beats of the tympany. These two sounds are so similar to the heart sounds as heard through a stethoscope or with an ear to the chest that the meaning of this movement is clear. One can feel the rhythm of the heart beating gently and contentedly in some passages and excitedly with anticipation in others. As each instrument takes up the theme, we sense that no heart beats alone, all beat in unison. The lyric third movement expresses, in my opinion, the longing for love that resides in the heart. This longing is fulfilled in the final movement where the chorus sings "The Ode to Joy." The vocal rendition transforms the symphony from an objective presentation to a subjective expression and translates the experience from the dramatic to the personal level. In this symphony Beethoven through his genius opened our hearts to joy and so brought joy to our hearts.

In its rhythmic activity, the heart is unique among the organs of the body. An isolated frog heart if perfused with blood and supplied with oxygen will continue to beat without nervous stimulation. A strip of heart muscle suspended in a physiological solution will also show spontaneous rhythmic contractions. This means that the rhythm of the heart is inherent in its tissue, the cardiac muscle. Within the organism, this inherent rhythm is regulated by several pacemakers who are, of course, under nervous control. Cardiac muscle is also unique in that it is a cross between the voluntary and the involuntary musculature. It has striations like the voluntary muscles but it is mediated by the autonomic nervous system and forms a sanctum which allows impulses to pass freely from one cell to another.

We use the expression, "Put your heart in it" to denote a total commitment to an activity. On this level, perhaps the deepest level one can feel, the movements of the body are sparked by a rhythm that emanates from the heart. The clearest example is the sexual function. There are two rhythmic patterns to the sexual movements, one voluntary and the other involuntary. During the first phase of coitus, the pelvic movements of both the man and the woman are consciously made and under ego control. At this stage the bodily excitation is relatively superficial although gradually deepening through the frictional contact and the pelvic swings. Breathing is still fairly quiet and the heart beat is only slightly accelerated.

When the excitation touches the internal organs a dramatic change occurs which ushers in the climax. In the man the seminal vesicle, the prostate and the urethra begin a pulsation that will culminate in the ejaculatory spurts of the semen. In the woman this is manifested in contractions of the uterus and the extended labia minora. If the excitations remain limited to the genital area only a partial orgasm occurs. If it spreads upward and reaches the heart the whole body goes into a convulsive type of reaction in which all voluntary control is surrendered to a primitive beat.

In the full orgasm, the pelvic movements which have been gradually increasing in frequency become involuntary and faster. Their rhythm becomes coordinated with the rhythm of the genital pulsations, the ejaculatory squirts in the man and the contractions of the labia minora in the woman. The breathing deepens and quickens to become part of this overall rhythm. The heart accelerates; its beat becomes conscious and one feels the pulse of life in every cell of the body.

Does the heart join in the total abandonment to pleasure or does it set the pace for the flight to orgasm and ecstasy? The question is not one I can answer at this time. The body is a unity that, we must remember, developed from a single cell. What is certain is that if the heart is not involved in the rhythm of the climax, the sexual experience will fall short of the highest bliss.

The ecstasy of orgasm is a bodily response to a sexual excitation that reaches and opens the heart. This concept is fully explored in Love and Orgasm. Love makes us feel lighthearted. The loss of a loved one makes the heart heavy with grief. I do not believe these are empty metaphors.

Every person in love has experienced the excitement in his heart. An excited heart is light, it leaps for joy. But it is not only the heart that leaps for joy. The lover skips and dances down the street. The rhythm of his heart dictates the movements of his whole body.

Notes

1. Reich, Wilhelm, *Function of the Orgasm*, New York, Orgone Institute Press, 1942, p. 257.
2. Feibleman, J.K., "A Philosophic Analysis of Pleasure" in *The Role of Pleasure in Behavior*, ed. R.G. Heath, New York: Harper & Row, 1964, p. 253.
3. Rado, Sandor, "Hedonic Self-Regulation" in *The Role of Pleasure in Behavior,* op. cit., p. 261.
4. Lowen, Alexander, *The Betrayal of the Body*, New York: MacMillan, 1967.

3

Breathing, Movement and Feeling: The Basis of Bioenergetic Analysis

LECTURE I: BREATHING

There are self-evident truths that need no demonstration. But, because they are self-evident they escape our attention. For example, no one will deny the importance of being alive. We want to be alive, yet we neglect to breathe, we are afraid to move, and we are reluctant to feel. Another self-evident truth is that personality is expressed through the body as much as through the mind. An individual cannot be divided into a mind and a body. Yet our studies of personality have concentrated on the mind to the relative neglect of the body.

The body of a person tells us much about his personality. His posture, the look in his eyes, the set of his jaw, the carriage of his head, and the position of his shoulders are only a few of the many indices of character to which we unconsciously react. There are other characteristics such as the quality of a handshake, the tone of the voice, and the spontaneity of gesture that impress us immediately. Since these bodily expressions identify a person, they can also be used in the diagnosis of personality disturbance.

The principles and practice of Bioenergetic Analysis rest upon the concept of a functional identity between the mind and body. This means that a change in personality is conditioned upon a change in the functions of the body. The two functions that are most important in this regard are *breathing* and *movement*. In the emotionally ill person both of these functions are disturbed by chronic muscular tensions. These tensions are the physical counterparts of psychological conflicts. Through these tensions, the conflicts become structured in the body as a restriction of breathing and a limitation of motility. Only by releasing these tensions, and resolving the conflicts, can there be a significant improvement in personality.

Breathing and movement determine *feeling*. An organism only feels the movements of its body. In the absence of movement there is no feeling. When, for example, an arm is immobilized, it becomes numb and the person loses the feeling of his arm. One has to restore its motility to recapture the feeling. The depth of respiration affects the intensity of feeling. By holding the breath, feeling can be reduced or deadened. Just as strong emotions stimulate breathing, the activation of respiration evokes suppressed feelings. Death is an arrest of respiration, a cessation of movement, and a loss of all feeling. To be wholly alive is to breathe deeply, move freely and feel fully. These self-evident truths cannot be ignored if we value life.

The importance of proper breathing to emotional and physical health is overlooked by most physicians and therapists. We know that breathing is necessary to life, that oxygen provides the energy to move the organism, but we do not realize that inadequate breathing reduces the vitality of the organism. The common complaints of tiredness and exhaustion are not generally attributed to poor breathing. Yet, depression and fatigue are direct results of a depressed respiration. The metabolic fires burn low in the absence of sufficient oxygen like a fire with a poor draft. Instead of glowing with life, the poor breather is cold, dull and lifeless. He lacks warmth and energy. His circulation is directly affected by a lack of oxygen. In chronic cases of poor breathing, the arterioles become constricted and the red blood count drops.

Most people are poor breathers. Their breathing is shallow and they have a strong tendency to hold their breath in any situation of stress. Even in such simple stress situations as driving a car, typing a letter, or waiting for an interview, people tend to limit their breathing. The result is to increase their tension. When people are made aware of breathing, they realize how often they hold their breath and how much they inhibit breathing. Patients commonly remark, "I notice how little I breathe."

I became aware of the relation between breathing and tension at college. As a member of the R.O.T.C., I participated in rifle practice at the local armory. My shooting was erratic, my aim was uneven. One of the professional officers watching me advised me, "Before you press the trigger, take three deep breaths. On the third breath let the air out slowly, and while doing so, squeeze the trigger gradually." I followed his advice and was amazed to find that my arm steadied and that I began to hit the bull's eye. This experience proved valuable in other situations. I used to sit in the dentist's chair in a state of tension, gripping the arms tightly. This not only increased my fear but, as I discovered subsequently, also augmented the pain. When I focused my attention upon my breathing instead, I was pleasurably surprised to find that not only was I less afraid but it seemed to hurt less. Breathing deeply had a similar relaxing effect upon my performance during examinations. By taking time to breathe I could also organize my thoughts better.

Many years later, in my professional practice, I realized that the restriction of breathing was directly responsible for the inability to concentrate and the restlessness that troubles many students. I am often consulted by parents about the difficulties their children have with school work. An examination of the child always revealed that his body was tense and his breathing minimal. The child became restless when he attempted to focus his attention for an extended period on a school book. His mind wandered. He felt compelled to move. He sat and struggled, but he could not study easily. Adults who do not breathe well have the same trouble. Their concentration and effectiveness are reduced.

The inability to breathe fully and deeply is also responsible for the failure to achieve full satisfaction in sex. Holding the breath at the approach of climax cuts off the strong sexual sensations. Normally, the breath is exhaled with the forward swing of the pelvis. If inhalation occurs during the forward movement, the diaphragm contracts and prevents the giving in necessary for orgastic release. Any restriction on breathing during the sexual act reduces the sexual pleasure.

Inadequate respiration produces anxiety, irritability and tension. It underlies such symptoms as claustrophobia and agoraphobia. The claustrophobic person feels that he cannot get enough air in an enclosed space. The agoraphobic person becomes frightened in open spaces because it stimulates his breathing. Every difficulty in breathing creates anxiety. If the difficulty is severe, it may lead to panic or terror.

Why do so many people have difficulty in breathing fully and easily? The answer is that breathing creates feelings and people are afraid to feel. They are afraid to feel their sadness, their anger and their fear. As children, they held their breath to stop crying, they drew back their shoulders and tightened their chests to contain their anger, and they constricted their throats to prevent screaming. The effect of each of these maneuvers is to limit and reduce respiration. Conversely, the suppression of any feeling results in some inhibition of respiration. Now, as adults, they inhibit their breathing to keep these feelings in repression. Thus, the inability to breathe normally becomes the main obstacle to the recovery of emotional health.

Broadly speaking, since repression cannot be lifted until full respiration is restored, it is important to understand the mechanisms that block breathing. I shall discuss two typical disturbances of respiration. In one the breathing is more or less confined to the chest, to the relative exclusion of the abdomen. In the second, the breathing is mainly diaphragmatic with relatively little movement in the chest. The first type of breathing is typical of the schizoid personality, the second of the neurotic personality.

In the schizoid individual, the diaphragm is immobilized and the abdominal muscles are tightly contracted. These tensions cut off sensations in the lower half of the body, especially the sexual feelings of the pelvis. The chest is held in the deflated position, and is generally narrow and constricted. Breathing-in, therefore, is limited and the result is inadequate oxygen and a lowered metabolism. Breathing-in is literally a sucking in of air and requires an aggressive attitude to the environment. However, aggression is reduced in the schizoid individual who is closed off emotionally from the world. He manifests an unconscious reluctance to breathe because he is fixated at the uterine level where his oxygen needs were met without his effort. To overcome the schizoid block to breathing-in, his terror must be released and his aggression mobilized. He must feel that he has a right to make demands on life, in the most primitive sense, to suck.

On the other hand, in the neurotic individual, where aggression is not as blocked as in the schizoid, the chest is immobilized while the diaphragm and upper abdomen are relatively free. The chest is generally held in an expanded position and the lungs contain a large amount of reserve air. The neurotic person finds it difficult to breathe out fully. He holds on to his reserve air as a security measure. Breathing out is a passive procedure, it is the equivalent of "letting go." Full expiration is a giving in, a surrender to the body. Letting go of the air is experienced as a letting go of control which the neurotic individual fears. The diaphragmatic respiration of the neurotic is a more effective type of breathing than the thoracic respiration of the schizoid. Diaphragmatic breathing provides maximum air for a minimal effort and is adequate for ordinary purposes. However, unless both the chest and the abdomen are engaged in the respiratory effort, the unity of the body is split and emotional responsiveness is limited.

Normal or healthy breathing has a unitary and total quality. Inspiration begins with an outward movement of the abdomen as the diaphragm contracts and the abdominal muscles relax. The wave of expansion then spreads upward to embrace the thorax. It is not cut off in the middle as in disturbed people. Expiration starts as a letting down in the chest and proceeds as a wave of contraction to the pelvis. It produces a sensation of flow along the front of the body which ends in the genitals. In healthy breathing the front of the body moves as one piece in a wave-like motion. This kind of breathing is seen in young children and animals whose emotions are not blocked. Such breathing actually involves the whole body, and tension in any part of the body disturbs this normal pattern. For example, pelvic immobility disrupts this pattern. Normally, there is a slight backward movement of the pelvis in inspiration and a slight forward movement in expiration. This is what Reich called the orgasm reflex. If the pelvis is locked in the forward or backward position, this balance wheel action of the pelvis is prevented.

The head is also actively involved in the breathing process. Together with the throat, it forms a great sucking organ which brings the air into the lungs. If the throat is constricted, this sucking action is reduced. When the air is not sucked in, the breathing is shallow. It has been observed in infants that any disturbance of their sucking impulse affects their breathing. I have observed that as soon as patients suck the air, their breathing becomes deeper.

The connection between sucking and breathing is clearly seen in cigarette smoking. The first drag on a cigarette is a strong sucking action which draws in the smoke as one would draw in air. There is a temporary feeling of satisfaction as the smoke fills the throat and lungs, and the person feels his lungs come alive in response to the irritant of the tobacco.

This use of the cigarette to excite the respiratory movements creates a dependence on the smoke. The first drag is followed by a second and a third, etc. Smoking then becomes a compulsion. The smoke itself has a depressing effect upon respiratory activity apart from its initial stimulation. The more a person smokes the less he breathes. However, because of his first experience, he cannot get away from the feeling that the cigarette is essential to help him breathe.

The function of smoking to stimulate breathing is seen in two situations, the morning cigarette and smoking under stress. The morning cigarette starts the day for some people but it also hangs them up on the cigarette the rest of the day. In situations of stress, the average person tends to hold his breath. This makes him anxious. To start breathing and overcome his anxiety, he takes a cigarette. Thus, a habit is established:

reach for a cigarette when under stress. The motto for compulsive smokers should be: take a breath instead of a puff.

Depth of breathing is measured by the length of the respiratory wave not by its amplitude. The deeper the breathing the more the wave extends into the lower abdomen. In truly deep breathing the respiratory movements reach and involve the floor of the pelvis and one can actually feel sensations in that area. The downward expansion of the lungs is limited by the diaphragm which separates the thorax from the abdomen. When we speak, therefore, of abdominal breathing we do not mean that any air penetrates the abdomen. Abdominal breathing describes the bodily movements in breathing. It denotes that the abdomen is actively engaged in the inspiratory process, its expansion and relaxation allow the diaphragm to descend. But of even greater importance is the fact that only through abdominal respiration does the wave of excitation associated with breathing embrace the whole body.

In my remarks above, I commented on the difference between schizoid breathing and neurotic breathing. The former is mostly confined to the thorax; the latter is mainly limited to the diaphragmatic area. Diaphragmatic breathing extends only into the upper part of the abdomen and thus while it is deeper than the more shallow breathing of the schizoid individual, it does not qualify as truly deep breathing. From this point of view the depth of breathing is a reflection of the emotional health of a person. The healthy person breathes with his whole body or, more specifically, his breathing movements extend deep down into his body. In a man, it could be said, broadly speaking, that he breathes into his "balls."

Breathing cannot be dissociated from sexuality. Indirectly, it provides the energy for the sexual discharge. The heat of passion is one aspect of the metabolic fires of which oxygen is an important element. Since the metabolic processes provide the energy for all living functions, the strength of the sexual drive is ultimately determined by these processes. Directly, the depth of respiration determines the quality of the sexual discharge. Unitary or total breathing, that is, a respiration that involves the whole body leads to an orgasm that includes the whole body. It is common knowledge that breathing is stimulated and its depth increased by sexual excitation. It is not generally recognized, however, that shallow or inadequate breathing reduces the level of sexual excitation. Restricted breathing prevents the spread of the excitation and keeps the sexual feeling localized in the genital area. Conversely, sexual inhibition, namely the fear of allowing sexual feelings to flood the pelvis and the body, is one of the causes of shallow and limited breathing. The respiratory wave normally flows from the mouth to the genital. In the upper end of the body it is connected to the erotic pleasure of sucking and nursing. In the lower end of the body it is tied to the sexual movements and sexual pleasure. Breathing is the basic pulsation (expansion and contraction) of the whole body; it is therefore, the foundation for the experience of pleasure and pain. Deep breathing is a sign that the organism experienced full erotic gratification in the oral stage and is capable of full sexual satisfaction in the genital stage.

Deep breathing charges the body and literally makes it come alive. And one of the self-evident truths about an alive body is that it looks alive: the eyes sparkle, the muscle tone is good, the skin has a bright color, and the body is warm. All this happens when a person breathes deeply.

Simple breathing exercises are ordinarily of little help in overcoming the problems associated with a disturbed respiration. The muscular tensions and the psychological conflicts that prevent deep breathing are not affected by such exercises. And the greater volume of inspired air which such exercises produce does not fully enter the blood stream and is not absorbed by the tissues. Only when the body feels the need for more oxygen and makes a spontaneous effort to breathe more deeply does a person become more alive through breathing. This is not to say that people should ignore the conscious component of breathing. We should try to be aware of the common tendency to hold our breath when under some stress and make an effort to breathe easily and deeply. By taking time to breathe we can counter to some extent the pressures that force us to keep going all the time.

Patients in bioenergetic therapy are encouraged to do special exercises which relax the muscular tensions of the body and stimulate its breathing. These exercises can also be recommended to the general public with a word of caution to the effect that they can release feelings or produce some anxiety. They will also promote a greater self-awareness, but in this process the person may feel pain in those parts of his body that were previously immobilized. This is especially true of the lower back. Neither the released feelings nor the anxiety or pain is any cause for alarm. These exercises should not be done compulsively nor pushed to an extreme since in themselves they will not solve the complicated personality problems that trouble most people.

Patients in therapy who do these special exercises designed to deepen breathing almost invariably develop tingling sensations in various parts of the body, the feet, the hands and the face, and very occasionally extending over the whole body. If the tingling sensations become intense, feelings of numbness and paralysis may also supervene. These sensations, known as *parasthesias* in medicine, are regarded as symptoms of the hyperventilation syndrome. Doctors interpret these symptoms as due to the discharge of too much carbon dioxide from the blood through intensive breathing. I don't believe this interpretation is fully accurate. Runners who breathe heavily do not develop these symptoms. I regard them as a sign that the person's body has become overcharged with oxygen which he is unable to utilize. He may also become dizzy because of this excess charge which disturbs his customary equilibrium. Both the dizziness and the parasthesias disappear when the breathing returns to normal.

As the patient's capacity to tolerate higher levels of excitation and oxygen charge increases, the parasthesias and dizziness diminish and disappear. The tingling is a superficial excitation which tends to deepen into specific feelings with continued work on the breathing. Sadness, longing and crying frequently emerge and reach expression. These, in turn, may give way to anger. Numbness and paralysis are indications of fear and contraction in the face of the increased excitation. These reactions, too, disappear as the patient's tolerance for feeling grows.

The basic bioenergetic breathing exercise is done by arching backwards over a rolled up blanket on a stool two feet high. This is shown in Figure 1.

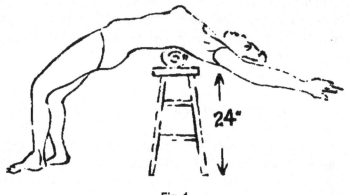

Fig. 1

When done at home the stool should be placed alongside a bed so the head and arms which are extended backward hang over or touch the bed. Since this is a stress position, the mouth should be open and the breathing allowed to develop freely and easily. Most people tend to hold their breath in this position as they do in most stress situations. This tendency must be consciously countered. The legs should be parallel, the feet resting flatly on the floor about 12 inches apart, and the pelvis should be allowed to hang freely. If this position induces some pain in the lower back it is an indication of tension in that area. If one relaxes to the position, the breathing will become deeper and fuller (more abdominal and of greater amplitude). The rolled up blanket is placed between the shoulder blades but this position can be varied to mobilize the different muscles of the back.

The position should not be held if it becomes too uncomfortable or if one feels choked. It is advisable that the beginner start slowly, and except in special circumstances, hold a stress position for no longer than two minutes. The purpose of this exercise is to promote one's breathing and not to test one's endurance.

The effectiveness of this exercise is shown by the fact that in many persons it will induce crying or a feeling of anxiety. I recall a case where a patient in her first experience with the stool developed panic. She had taken several deep breaths when suddenly she was on her feet gasping for air. A moment later she burst into sobs and her panic disappeared. The deep breathing for which she was unprepared opened a feeling of sadness which welled up in her throat. Unconsciously, her throat closed as she tried to choke the feeling off and she could not breathe. This was the only time I saw a patient react in this way to the exercise but it indicates the potential power of the exercise.

I use this exercise regularly to further my own breathing and to relax the tension between my shoulders. I keep a stool in my bedroom and get over it most mornings before breakfast. It helps overcome the tendency to round the shoulders and hunch forward which is found in most people. The exercise itself is the development of the natural tendency to stretch backward over the back of a chair which many people do spontaneously after they have been sitting hunched forward for some time. All animals stretch upon arising and this exercise is a most effective form of stretching. After lying over the stool for a minute or so and breathing deeply, I reverse the position with another exercise.

In this second exercise the person bends forward to touch the ground with his finger tips. His feet are about 12 inches apart, the toes slightly turned inward and the knees slightly bent. There should be no weight on the hands; the whole weight of the body rests on the legs and feet. The head hangs down as loose as possible. The weight of the body should fall midway between the heel and ball of the foot. This position is illustrated in Figure 2.

We use this position in bioenergetic therapy to bring a person into a feeling of contact with his legs and feet. At the same time, it stimulates abdominal respiration by relaxing the front wall of the body, especially the abdominal musculature which was stretched by the first exercise. Again the mouth should be open and the breathing allowed to develop easily and freely. If a person holds his breath in any exercise, the value is lost.

When this exercise is done correctly the legs should begin to vibrate or tremble and they will continue to vibrate as long as the breathing continues, sometimes even increasing in intensity. This vibration is normal. All alive bodies vibrate in stress positions as will be explained in the next lecture.

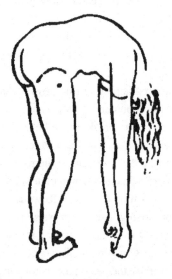

Fig. 2

Normally, breathing is an involuntary rhythmic activity of the body under the control of the vegetative nervous system. It is also subject to conscious control so that the person can deliberately increase or decrease the rate and depth of his respiration. Conscious breathing, however, does not influence the typical involuntary pattern of respiration which is closely tied to the emotional responsiveness of the individual. The involuntary vibrations of the body, on the other hand, have an immediate affect on the respiratory pattern. The vibrations of the legs and other parts of the body stimulate and release the breathing movements. When a body is in a state of vibration, breathing deepens spontaneously. This is because the vibratory state of a body is a manifestation of its emotional responsiveness.

Breathing is also directly involved in voice production, which is another vibratory activity of the body. Inhibitions in crying, screaming and yelling are structured in tensions which restrict respiration. The child who has been taught that "children are to be seen but not heard" does not breathe freely. The natural tendency to speak up, cry out or scream is choked off by spasms in the musculature of the neck. These tensions affect the quality of the voice, producing a speaking voice that is either too thin, too low, too flat or too sibilant. The voice must be restored to its full range and the specific neck tensions released if the breathing is to recover its full depth. The role of sound in bioenergetic analysis will be discussed in a subsequent lecture series.

LECTURE II: MOVEMENT

Several years ago a book was published entitled *The Myth of Mental Illness*. At last! I thought the psychiatric profession was beginning to realize that the term "mental illness" is a misnomer. I ordered the book and could hardly wait for its arrival. To my surprise, the thesis of the book, written by an eminent psychiatrist, was that these patients were not ill at all. He attempted to prove that the hysterical patients upon whom Freud founded his psychoanalytic concepts were malingerers. He claimed that they were pretending or that they were playing a game by rules different from those which guided normal people.

Recently, another book has become very popular, entitled *The Games People Play*. The argument of this book is that people play games to avoid intimacy. The different games are analyzed to show the ego motives which impel them. This idea of game playing is not new. It was most clearly stated in the term of one-up-manship. The person who analyzes the game, including the psychiatrist, is one-up on the person who is playing the game. But analyzing games becomes a new game and so nothing is gained.

It is interesting to speculate on why psychiatry has taken this turn. I think it reflects a deep feeling of discouragement in the general public, as well as among psychiatrists, with psychoanalytic thinking which has failed to provide people with the understanding and help so urgently needed. In desperation, people search anywhere for answers, not realizing that they are clutching at straws. The desperate person has neither the time nor the patience for a careful working out of his problems. He runs with the crowd like a person in a panic.

It is true that people play games in the sense that they have adopted certain roles in life which they are trying to fulfill. This is true of all my patients. These roles are not conscious. They are determined by attitudes which developed in childhood as a way of meeting the demands of parents. But a role is not a game in the real sense of the word game.

A game is a limited activity, whereas an unconscious role continues all the time. Such a role is a limitation of freedom, a fixed pattern of behavior which is imposed on the personality. The role is manifested in the carriage and movement of the body. To step out of a role one must change the way one moves and breathes.

Mental illness is a misnomer. People suffer from emotional disturbances. The word *emotion* is composed of the prefix "e" and the stem "motion." Emotion means to move out. An emotional disturbance is an inability to move out towards people and the world. By definition, one can say that emotional conflicts distort or limit the motility of the body. They impede movement outward. Similarly, any disturbance in the ability of an organism to move out denotes an emotional conflict. One can, therefore, determine emotional conflicts in a person from the way he moves.

The quality of a person's movement is studied from two points of view, spontaneity and control. Spontaneity is a function of self-expression. The more alive a person is the more spontaneous are his movements. The body is naturally expressive; it is constantly changing to reflect its inner feelings. In this respect, it is like a flame which is never the same at any two moments. While a body is more structured than a flame, it is not as rigid as a machine. It has a fluid quality and responds to the play of the inner forces.

Normally, control represents the ego's restraint upon spontaneity and is designed to produce more effective action. Through ego control the spontaneous motility of the body is channeled and integrated to achieve a desired goal. A healthy ego control does not diminish the body's spontaneity. When control and spontaneity are integrated in the body's movement, the result is coordination. Coordination reflects the degree to which the ego is identified with the body and yet is in command of its movements. A healthy person is well coordinated in his movements, he is spontaneous and yet in control.

Emotional illness is characterized either by a loss of spontaneity or a deficiency of ego control, or both. Broadly speaking, the emotionally disturbed person moves compulsively or impulsively. The compulsive person is rigid, his ego restraints are so severe that his movements take on a mechanical, patterned quality, and spontaneity is missing. In the impulsive person the ego control is weakened and impulses break through in a hysterical manner. The impulsive person is hyperactive; he can neither sit still nor channel his energy into constructive activities. His inadequate ego is constantly being overwhelmed by his feelings. At the same time he is constantly frustrated since his feelings spill out without achieving anything.

The compulsive person is afraid to let go of his rigid control, the impulsive person is unable to maintain control. In effect, the impulsive person is discharging his energy wildly to avoid the feelings in his body. He becomes irritable to avoid feeling his anger, hysterical to avoid feeling his sadness, and promiscuous to avoid his sexual feelings. He runs before he is afraid, cries before he is hurt, and attacks before he is threatened. He behaves like an infant and his movements, like those of an infant, are uncoordinated and ineffective.

Characterological rigidity is manifested on both the psychic and physical levels, but is always expressed in bodily terms. We say of a person that he is stiff-necked, poker-faced, tight-lipped, unbending, grim-jawed, etc. Rigidity stems from the holding back of feelings. A person stiffens to hold back his anger, he sets his jaw not to be afraid, and he tightens his abdomen not to cry. To suppress feeling, chronic muscular tensions develop which impart a rigidity to the body.

The impulsive person is not free from such tensions either. In the compulsive person the muscular tensions are predominantly longitudinal, which stiffens the body. In the impulsive person, they are annular or horizontal, which segments the body. However, these distinctions are a matter of degree. Tensions of both kinds are found in all disturbed persons.

The loss of spontaneity and control also produces a condition of flaccidity which is both physical and psychic. We describe such persons as spineless or weak-kneed, etc. We may say of a person that he cannot hold his head up. Flaccidity denotes the denial of feeling. The surrender or denial of feeling produces a collapse of the peripheral musculature. In contrast, the rigid person holds back his feelings (contains them), whereas the impulsive person "acts them out" irresponsibly. The hysterical nature of impulsive behavior derives from the fact that while part of the body releases an impulse, another part resists the release.

Healthy emotional expressions never take the form of hysterical outbursts. They are ego syntonic, that is the feeling is expressed with the full support of the ego. As a result, the movement which expresses the feeling is unified and total. The corollary is also true. When a movement embraces the whole body in a unified way, the result is an emotional expression which the person feels. This principle underlies bioenergetic therapy.

Bioenergetic therapy aims at the restoration of the natural spontaneity of the body and the development of adequate ego control. It starts with breathing since the restriction of breathing limits the energy needed for movement and imposes a major restraint upon the body's motility. The respiratory waves (breathing in and breathing out) are the basic pulsatory movements of the body. As these waves pass through the body they activate the entire muscular system. The spontaneity of the body is guaranteed by the free movement of these waves. This means that as long as the respiration is uninhibited and deep there are no functional blocks to the flow of feeling. However, the release of tension cannot be achieved by breathing alone.

In all persons, as the breathing deepens, vibrations are set up in the body. These generally start in the legs but if they become strong enough, they can extend to and embrace the whole body. The vibrations may seem so strong that the patient feels he is going "to fall apart." The fear of "falling apart" is the physical counterpart of the fear of letting go. No one literally falls apart nor do one's defenses crumble though they are shaken by the experience. Through the vibration of the body the person becomes aware of the powerful forces that are immobilized in his body by muscular tension.

A healthy personality is a vibrant personality and a healthy body is a pulsating and vibrating body. In a state of health the vibrations are relatively fine and steady like the hum of a smooth running automobile. When all vibrations cease in a body, it goes dead like a car when the motor stops. Individuals whose bodies do not vibrate are emotionally dead. On the other hand, a body that shakes too violently is similar to a car whose spark plugs are fouled, valves corroded and bearings dry. As these bugs are ironed out in a car its vibration becomes a purr. When the body of a human being purrs, it has an animal's freedom of movement.

These "bugs" in the body of a person are chronic muscular tensions. They develop as an inhibition of movement and can only be discharged through the release of the movement. Each tense muscle is a contracted muscle which has to be stretched to activate its potential for movement. Since the muscle is an elastic tissue, the active stretching of spastic muscles will often set them into vibration ranging all the way from fine fibrillations to gross shaking. The vibration regardless of its quality serves to loosen the chronic spasticity of the muscle.

Have you noticed how a baby's chin quivers just before it starts to cry? This quiver is the start of the larger vibration that is crying. It sometimes happens with patients that when the bodily vibration reaches the chest and throat the patient breaks into sobs. I have also seen it happen, when the patient was prone with legs extended upwards, that the vibrations of the legs changed into spontaneous kicking movements.

The position in which the legs are made to vibrate easily is illustrated below. The person lies on a bed with legs extended upward, knees slightly bent and the feet in extreme flexion. If an upward thrust is maintained in the heels with the pelvis resting on the bed, the legs will begin to tremble involuntarily. From this position spontaneous kicking movements sometimes develop. The feet are about 6 inches apart.

In addition to the involuntary movements which form the base of the work with the body, a number of expressive movements are used to mobilize and release the suppressed feelings. These start as voluntary movements but they can become involuntary to some degree if the emotion evoked becomes strong enough to take over the movement.

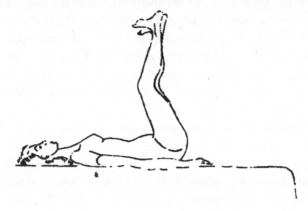

Fig. 3

One of the simplest exercises used for this purpose is kicking the bed while lying flat on it. The legs are held outstretched and are kicked up and down in a rhythmic manner. If the body is free, the person's breathing will become synchronized with the kicking. This will not occur if the upper half of the body is held stiffly. In this exercise, the head will be whipped up and down with each kick as the body gives in to the movements. If coordination is disturbed, the head will not move at all or move side to side while the legs are moving up and down.

Kicking is an expressive movement. To kick is to protest, and every person has something to protest or kick about. Therefore, it is a movement that everyone should be able to do with feeling. If a person's self-expression has been blocked by his parents, his kicking will have an impotent quality. Continued work with this exercise and others will generally release the blocks and permit the expression of convincing movements.

To make the kicking more meaningful the person is directed to express an appropriate feeling in words. He can say "No" or "I won't" or, what is even more meaningful, "Leave me alone." These utterances should be made in a loud and forceful tone while the legs are kicked forcibly into the bed. The use of sound and words with this movement integrates the ego attitude with the bodily expression and thus promotes coordination and control. When a person lets himself go fully in sound and movement to the feeling, the kicking becomes more rapid while the voice may rise to the level of a scream. At this point the emotion envelops the whole body and is sharply experienced by the person. Yet no matter how intense the feeling, the person is fully aware of what he is doing and can stop the expression at will.

A similarly expressive movement can be made using the arms. In this exercise the person also lies on the bed but his knees are bent and his feet are flat. With fists clenched, both arms are raised over the head and brought down hard alongside of the body in a blow. At the same time the person is encouraged to say "No" or "I won't." The movement is repeated a number of times while the person tries to get a convincing tone in his voice and an effective blow with his arms. It is surprising how difficult this is to achieve. The voice often has an undertone of pleading, crying or fear while the blows are mechanical or powerless. If one challenges the patient while he is doing this exercise by saying "You will," the intensity of the expressed feeling can often be gauged. Some patients stop and others change their statement to "I will." A few accept the challenge and confront the therapist with an intensified, "I won't."

These movements not only arouse feeling but they stimulate the breathing and set the body in vibration. This happens to the degree that the patient can allow himself to experience and express a negative and hostile feeling. Any holding against the feeling will be manifested by a lack of coordination or gracelessness in the movements. This is especially evident when the patient tries to execute a temper tantrum reaction. In this exercise the legs are drummed into the bed with bent knees while the arms flail the bed alternately. When this movement is executed correctly, the right arm and the right leg move synchronously and alternate with the left arm and left leg. The head rotates to the side that is making the striking movement. When the movement is uncoordinated, the rhythm of the leg movements differs from that of the arm movements or there is a crossing phenomenon: the left arm moves downward with the right leg and the right arm moves with the left leg, not infrequently the head turns in the opposite direction to the movement. Uncoordinated movements leave the person with a feeling of dissatisfaction.

Another procedure in the therapy is to get the patient to hit the bed with his fists or a tennis racquet from a standing position. The movement expresses anger but most patients doing this exercise at the beginning of the therapy do not feel anything while executing the movements. Girls may even say, "It's silly." One observes that the sense of "no meaning" accompanies a movement that is awkward. An awkward movement feels silly. Similarly a movement that is done mechanically evokes no feeling. However, as soon as the whole body participates in the activity with coordinated movements, the feeling of anger arises.

It cannot be over-emphasized that emotional expression is a function of unified and coordinated movement. When a patient develops coordination, he gains control over his behavior. He is not a controlled individual as is the compulsive person nor is he an impulsive individual who cannot adapt his behavior to the situation. At the same time he is spontaneous because the motility of his body is unrestricted.

In the above exercises I described how bioenergetic therapy works with the aggressive movements which express negativity, hostility and anger. It is equally important to develop the same unity and coordination in the expression of tenderness, affection and desire. This is done by using movements of reaching out with the mouth and arms. In most persons these expressive movements are constricted by muscular spasticities in the jaw, throat and shoulders. In the presence of such tensions the expressive movements are awkward and hesitant. The person feels insecure and uncertain when he tries to make such movements. And since an awkward movement generally evokes an ambiguous response, the person making such an uncoordinated movement feels inadequate and rejected. What we call self-confidence is the awareness by an individual that he can express himself fully and freely in any situation by appropriate and graceful movements.

The person whose movements are not restricted by chronic muscular tensions has a natural grace. Gracefulness results when spontaneity and control are fully integrated. Stiffness and awkwardness are the signs of tension which interfere with the natural motility of the body. To remove these tensions one must become aware of them and understand their meaning.

LECTURE III: FEELING

It is an axiom of bioenergetic analysis that a person can only feel his body. One cannot feel the environment except through its effect upon the body. In reality, then, one feels how one's body reacts to the environment or to external objects and the perception of this feeling is projected upon the stimulus. Thus, when I sense that your hand is warm as it rests on my arm, what I am feeling is the warmth in my body as it is affected by your hand. All our feelings are body perceptions. How much we feel and how deeply we feel is a function of self-awareness.

Self-awareness means an awareness of the body. The individual who is aware of himself is in contact with his body. He senses what is going on in every part of his body; he is, in other words, in touch with himself. He feels the flow of sensation in his body associated with breathing, that is, he has streaming sensations in his body. But he also feels his tensions and constrictions for no one is free from such tensions. The person who lacks this self-awareness suffers from self-consciousness because he, too, is dimly aware that something is amiss which he does not understand. He feels awkward and ill at ease and his self-possession is diminished although he may make every conscious effort to hide this dim perception of himself.

In the unaware person there are areas of the body that lack sensation and are, therefore, missing from consciousness. For example, people are generally unaware of the expression on their faces. They do not know if they look sad, angry or disgusted. Some faces have such an obvious expression of pain that the observer is surprised that the person is unaware of it. Other areas of the body of which people are commonly unaware are the legs, the buttocks, the back and the shoulders. Every person knows that he has legs, buttocks, back and shoulders, but he doesn't feel them as alive parts of his body. He cannot tell whether his legs are relaxed or contracted, whether his buttocks are retracted or tucked forward, whether his back is up or down, and whether his shoulders are raised or lowered.

Such a lack of awareness means that the person has lost the full scope of the function of those parts of the body which are missing from consciousness. The person who doesn't feel his legs lacks a sense of security because he doesn't have the inner conviction that his legs will hold him up. He is not emotionally secure on his own feet and feels the need for someone or something to support him. The buttocks function as counterweights to maintain the normal, erect posture. When the buttocks are pulled forward, the upper half of the body tends to collapse. This can only be prevented by extruding the chest and stiffening the back. The tucked in buttocks resemble the posture of a dog with its tail between its legs. The individual who carries himself in this posture has lost his natural cockiness which can only be compensated then by an exaggerated ego pose based on rigidity. On the other hand, if the buttocks are retracted, the person loses the ability to swing his pelvis forward in a sexually aggressive manner. His body reveals a lordosis which is an exaggerated hollow in the small of the back. He suffers from sexual inadequacy because of an inability to discharge his sexual feeling.

Normally, the pelvis is suspended freely and moves spontaneously forward and back with the breathing. This movement is intensified in intercourse and results in the involuntary movements of the orgasm. The backward movement charges the pelvis with sensation and feeling while the forward movement discharges the feeling to the genitals. Chronic pelvic tensions which restrict pelvic motility reduce a person's orgastic potency. The sad thing about these tensions is that they decrease a person's awareness so that he doesn't know what is wrong with his sexual function. He may blame himself or his partner without any understanding of the cause of his difficulties.

Because of chronic tensions, the average person has little feeling in his back. One commonly finds that the back is either so rigid as to be unbending or so pliable as to offer no support for the body. In both cases, the person loses the ability to "back up his feelings" or to hold them back. Too much rigidity leads to compulsiveness, too great a flaccidity to impulsiveness. Lacking sensation in his back, he cannot mobilize his anger to overcome his frustrations. In an animal like a dog or a cat, one can literally see the back rise when the animal is angry. Even the hair along its back stands up as this part of his body is charged with feeling. Disturbed human beings become irritable or go into a rage but lack the animal ability to express anger in a direct way.

The tension in the back is generally associated with tensions which immobilize the shoulders. Two important functions are affected by shoulder tensions. One is the ability to reach out and the other is the ability to strike out. When the shoulders are fixed in a raised position the person is "hung up" as if he were suspended by a clothes hanger. Raised shoulders are an expression of fear. The shoulders go up in fright. The person with raised shoulders is hung up by his fear and is unable to let down. He is also hung up by his inability to reach out or strike out.

The unaware person is also unwary. His image of himself does not coincide with the picture he presents to others and his naive acceptance of this image leaves him open to unexpected responses. The person who thinks he presents a manly appearance because his chest is inflated is shocked when he learns that other people can see this as a pose. By the same token he is easily fooled by the poses and facades which other people erect. Only to the degree that you are aware of yourself are you aware of others, and only to the extent that you feel yourself as a person can you feel for another person.

The loss of self-awareness is caused by chronic muscle tension. This tension differs from the normal tensions of living by the fact that it is a persistent unconscious muscular spasticity that has become part of the body's structure or way of being. Because of this fact the person is unaware that he has such chronic tensions until they begin to cause him pain. When this happens he may sense the underlying tension but he has no awareness of what it means and why it developed. And he is completely helpless to do anything to relieve the tension. In the absence of pain, however, most people are completely oblivious to the way in which they hold themselves or move. They feel comfortable in their structured attitudes unaware of the limitations which these attitudes impose upon their potential for living.

A muscle becomes tense only under stress. When it is moving easily, the body feels no strain. Stresses are of two kinds, physical or emotional. Supporting a heavy weight is a physical stress, as is the continuation of a movement or activity when the muscle is tired. The person feels the pain of the tension, and stops the activity or drops the weight. If, however, there is no way to remove the stress, the muscle will go into spasm. An emotional stress is just like a physical one, the muscles are charged with a feeling that they cannot release. They contract to hold or contain the feeling just as they do to support a weight and if the feeling persists long enough, the muscle will go into spasm since it cannot get rid of the tension.

Any emotion which cannot be released is a stress for the muscles. This is true because an emotion is a charge which presses outward for release. A few examples will illustrate these ideas. Sadness or hurt feelings are released through crying. If the crying is inhibited because of parental objections or for other reasons, the muscles which normally react in crying become tense. These are the muscles of the mouth, throat, chest and abdomen. If the feeling which cannot be released is one of anger, the muscles of the back and shoulders become tense. Inhibited biting impulses lead to jaw tensions, inhibited kicking impulses to leg tensions. The correlation between muscle tension and inhibition is so exact that one can tell what impulses or feelings are inhibited in a person from a study of his muscular tensions.

As far as the muscle is concerned there is little difference between an external stress and an internal stress. Both place the muscle under tension. Physical stresses are generally conscious and tend to be of shorter duration than emotional stresses, which are often unconscious and tend to persist.

When a muscle goes into spasm, it contracts and stays contracted until the stress is removed. You will find this to be true of a leg cramp, for instance. To get rid of the cramp, you must change your position and move the cramped muscle. A cramp, however, is a very acute tension which allows no alternative. The tensions that arise through inhibition are chronic tensions which develop slowly, through repeated experiences and so insidiously that the person is hardly conscious of the tension. Even if he is conscious of the tension, he knows no way to release it. He has to live with it, and the only way to live with a tension is to forget about it.

Since mind and body are one, the unconscious must have a physical meaning. The unconscious is that part of the body which is not perceived. It is important to know that a nerve and its muscle form one fundamental unit. When a muscle is chronically contracted, the effector nerve to the muscle is isolated from the total nerve network as far as voluntary movements are concerned. The repression of a feeling occurs when the muscle that is charged with the feeling is cut off from awareness by chronic tension and the nerve to this muscle is isolated from the nerve grid. For example, the traumatic experiences of toilet training are repressed in those persons who have no awareness of their anal tensions. To bring these memories back from the unconscious, the person has to gain contact with the muscles of his pelvic floor.

Self-awareness is dependent on movement. We perceive that which moves; that which doesn't move fades from consciousness. Thus, any part of the body which is immobile because of chronic tension is removed from perception. The individual is not even aware of the tension. The first step in restoring self-awareness is to become conscious of tension. This is done by putting a person in positions in which he feels his tensions. He is also asked to execute certain movements in which his coordination is tested. When a person has gained some contact with the deadened areas of his body, he is in a position to release the chronic tensions that underlie the deadness.

A relaxed muscle is a muscle charged with energy. It is like a loaded gun ready for firing. The trigger which discharges the muscle is an impulse from its effector nerve. The discharge of the muscle produces a contraction which is translated into movement. A contracted muscle cannot move until it's recharged with new energy. This energy is brought to the muscle in the form of oxygen and sugar. Without a supply of additional energy, it is impossible to release contracted muscles. The important factor in this process is oxygen since without sufficient oxygen, the metabolic process in the muscle comes to a halt. This fact points up the importance of breathing for relaxation and for the lifting of repressions. When a patient's breathing is deepened, his tense muscles will go into spontaneous vibration like a spring which has been released from tension.

In some patients, the vibrations may turn into spontaneous expressive movements as the body itself releases its repressed impulses. Generally, movements are started consciously and the repressed impulses are evoked when the movements take on a total quality. A patient may begin by kicking the couch as an exercise, but as he lets go to the movement, it takes over the whole body producing an emotional release. Tense muscles can only be released by expressive movements, that is, movements in which the activity expresses the feeling. As long as a movement is mechanically performed, the repressed impulses are held back.

What role does analysis play in bioenergetic therapy? The emphasis in this discussion has been on the physical aspects of this therapy and this may give a reader the impression that the analytic understanding of character plays a secondary role. This, of course, is not true. It is as important for a patient to know the origin of his conflicts as it is for him to gain self-awareness through bodily activity. The two approaches must be attuned to each other for an effective therapy. All the modalities of psychotherapy and psychoanalysis are used in bioenergetic therapy to further self-understanding and self-expression. This includes the interpretation of dreams and the working through of the transference situation. In contrast to other forms of therapy the body is the foundation upon which the ego functions of self-understanding and self-expression are erected.

The basic bioenergetic concept is that each chronic muscle tension pattern must be dealt with on three levels: (1) its history or origin in the infantile or childhood situation, (2) its present-day meaning in terms of the individual's character, and (3) its effect upon bodily functioning. Only this holistic view of the phenomenon of muscle tension can produce those changes in the personality that can have a lasting value. This leads to several important propositions.

1. Every chronically tense muscle group represents an emotional conflict which is unresolved and probably repressed. The tension results from an impulse seeking expression that meets a restraint based on fear. A jaw tension may represent the conflict between an impulse to bite and the fear that such action would lead to punitive measures by the parent. The same tension could also be related to an impulse to cry and the fear that it will provoke the parent's anger or rejection. Tensions have multiple determinations since all parts of the body are involved in every emotional expression. This means that every tension must be worked through in terms of all the movements in which the tense muscle can participate. If possible, the specific conflicts involving the tense muscle group should become conscious both as to the impulse it holds and the fear it denotes.

2. Every chronically tense muscle represents a negative attitude. Every inhibition is perceived as a constraint which leads to a feeling of hostility because of the loss of freedom. Therefore, before the impulse locked in the contracted muscle can be released, the negative feeling must be expressed as a general attitude. Feelings that have to be inhibited are mostly negative, hostile or sexual feelings. Parents do not encourage the expression of hostile feelings and, in most cases, they prohibit such expressions. These feelings are, then, generally repressed.

The generalized negative attitude expressed in the holding action of tense muscles extends to and includes the therapist and the therapeutic situation. It is covered by a facade of politeness and cooperation. One can get through this facade by the painstaking analysis of the transference or move immediately by making the expression of negativity the first order of business in therapy. Every patient in bioenergetic therapy confronts his concealed negativity by working with the expression of hostility and negativity physically and vocally.

The biological aspect of muscle tension is its relation to breathing, moving and feeling. These have been discussed above. Since every tension cuts down on sexual feeling, each patient becomes aware of how these tensions affect his sexual functioning.

Self-awareness or the sense of identity is dependent on the ability to say "No!" The assertion of the No demarcates the individual from his environment and asserts his individuality, vis a vis others. The person who can say "no" can say "yes." The person who can't say "no" is submissive and resentful. The ability to say "no" depends upon the inner freedom from restraint or freedom from chronic muscle tension. Every chronic muscle tension is a limitation upon self-assertion and self-awareness. These concepts are more fully explored in my book, *The Betrayal of the Body.*

4

Self-Expression
New Developments in Bioenergetic Therapy

LECTURE 1: SELF-EXPRESSION AND SPONTANEITY

The announcement of the 1968 series of public lectures described them as *New Developments in Bioenergetic Therapy*. These new developments included a special emphasis upon movement, the voice and the eyes. In the course of the lectures, it became apparent to me that each lecture dealt with a major modality of self-expression. A person expresses himself largely through his movements, his voice and his eyes. Although the function of self-expression was not specifically discussed during these lectures, it is, nevertheless, the theme that underlies these new developments in bioenergetic therapy.

Self-expression denotes the activity of a self and is, like self-preservation, an inherent quality of all living organisms. To be alive is to be expressive in form, movement, color, voice, etc. Adolf Portmann, a leading biologist, makes the statement in his fascinating book, *New Paths in Biology*, that "A rich inner life...depends largely on...that degree of inner independence, that degree of self-hood, which goes hand in hand with a rich manner of self-expression." To my mind, this says that the sense of identity or the degree of self-hood can be correlated with the range and variety, the richness of one's self-expression.

The Voice of the Body

A human being expresses himself both consciously and unconsciously. Every aspect of the body is an unconscious expression of the person-size, shape, tone, carriage, color of skin, hair and eyes. All of these plus other bodily manifestations give us a picture of the person which defines him at the moment in our minds. These are not static manifestations, for bodies are constantly changing. In addition, a person expresses himself through a myriad of spontaneous movements, utterances and looks. And superimposed upon these two levels there are the deliberate actions—willed movements, vocal statements and determined glances that express the self.

In this discussion I shall focus upon the level of spontaneous expressions since these are most directly connected with feelings.

In his paper "The Creative Attitude," Abraham Maslow says: "Full spontaneity is a guarantee of honest expression of the nature and the style of the freely functioning organism, and of its uniqueness. Both words, spontaneity and expressiveness, imply honesty, naturalness, truthfulness, lack of guile, non-imitativeness, etc., because they also imply a non-instrumental nature of the behavior, a lack of willful 'trying,' a lack of effortful striving or straining, a lack of interference with the flow of the impulses and the free 'radioactive' expression of the deep person."

If spontaneous behavior is compared with learned behavior, its relation to self-expressiveness is clear. Learned behavior generally reflects what one has been taught and must be regarded, therefore, as an expression of the teacher and not the self. A spontaneous gesture is a direct expression of an impulse, and therefore it is a direct manifestation of the inner self.

The current emphasis upon self-expression and spontaneity is part of the anti-intellectual and anti-rational movement that is taking place today. Among young people this movement is manifested in an identification with violence as a form of self-expression, in the rejection of established modes of dress and behavior, and in a new sexual freedom. Among more mature people it is expressed in the importance given to experience and learning as opposed to teaching and logic, in the recognition of feeling as a determinant of behavior, and in the respect accorded to the animal and by extension to man's animal nature.

For more than two thousand years man has striven to suppress his animal nature, to curb his instincts and to control his feelings. He has developed a civilization whose technological achievements are a tribute to the power of his mind. But in the process he has undermined his identity and lost his sense of self. He has become harnessed to the economic machine and reduced to being like a machine. He has subverted his energy to conquering nature, but he has destroyed his own soul. And he has lost the capacity for joy.

In his dilemma, he is finding that the rational therapies such as psychoanalysis are of little help. Purely verbal therapies are proving impotent to restore his sense of self and his freedom of self-expression. The non-rational aspect of life is in the body, not the mind. It is through his body that a person can recover the freedom of self-expression which is the conscious experience of the self.

Movement and Feeling

A feeling is the perception of a movement within the body. If nothing moves within the body, there is no feeling. Thus a dead man has no feelings because all internal movement has ceased in his body. Similarly, the displacement of a body in space does not create any feelings unless it provokes some internal movement. Children love to swing because of the pleasurable internal sensations that are produced by this motion. If an internal movement is not perceived, there is no feeling. One doesn't ordinarily feel the beating of his heart. However, if the heart's action is unusual and reaches consciousness, one will have a feeling. One can actually feel the heart leap with joy or open with love or contract with fear, if one's self-awareness is undisturbed.

We experience emotions only when the internal movements of the body embrace the totality of the body. A limited or restricted movement lacks an emotional quality. If the knee jerks, one will feel the movement but it will lack an emotional tone. We say that we are moved to tears, or to anger, or laughter, etc. We cannot evoke these emotions deliberately. They are not subject to the will. They are states of possession. We are possessed by a force within us that moves us to cry, to laugh, to be angry or to be afraid. The word *emotion* means to move outward—to move in an expressive way, not by direction of the mind but as an action of the self.

A living body is never completely at rest. There are constant internal movements which vary in quality and intensity according to the state of excitation. These internal movements constitute the motility of an organism. The greater its motility the more expressive it is. When its motility is reduced, its degree of self-expression is limited.

The motility of a body is directly affected by the energy level of the body. It takes energy to maintain a state of motion. When a body's energy is low or depleted, its motility is necessarily decreased. A direct line, therefore, connects

energy→motility →feeling→spontaneity→self-expression.

This sequence also operates in reverse. If an individual's self-expression is blocked, his spontaneity is reduced. This reduction of spontaneity lowers the feeling tone which, in turn, decreases the motility of the body and depresses its energy level. I shall discuss each of these functions in order starting with energy.

Energy, Movement and Feeling

Albert Szent-Gyorgi, the Nobel Prize-winning physiologist, said it takes energy to move the wheels of life. This energy is provided by the metabolic processes of the body. Part of the food we eat, especially the sugars and fats, are oxidized by the body to yield energy. This process involves the consumption of oxygen. It has been the practice to measure the basal metabolic rate by the intake of oxygen during conditions of rest. Breathing is a valid yardstick to gauge the energy level of a person. In general, if the breathing is shallow, the energy level is low. Deeper breathing goes hand in hand with more energy. It is common experience that increasing the draft of a fire raises the intensity of the fire and produces more energy.

The connection between breathing, energy and feeling may be stated as follows: When one becomes excited, one breathes more deeply. When one breathes more deeply, one becomes excited. The depth of feeling is roughly proportional to the depth of the respiration. In bioenergetic therapy we start with the function of breathing because this is the most direct way to increase the energy level of the organism. We try to get a patient to breathe thoracically, diaphragmatically and abdominally so that the respiratory wave moves through the body from head to foot.

Breathing is also directly related to the motility of the body. One cannot breathe freely if chronic muscular tensions block the movement of the wave. If the chest is unyielding, breathing becomes diaphragmatic. If the abdomen is constricted, breathing tends to be limited to the upper half of the body. As the patient breathes more deeply, the body becomes energized and the respiratory wave gains momentum and breaks through the tensions. One immediate effect of deep breathing is to set the body in vibration.

The vibration generally starts in the legs but it can extend upward to include the whole body. At first the patient may be surprised, startled or a little frightened, but it has such a releasing effect that it is soon desired. The vibrations may be coarse or fine depending on the degree of charge and amount of tension in the body. When the tension is severe, the deep breathing will produce such strong vibrations that the patient may feel he is shaking apart. The vibrations have the effect of shaking the body loose from its chronic tensions and thus increasing the motility of the body. As the tensions decrease, the vibrations become finer and more coordinated until the body hums like a smoothly functioning machine. One cannot have a vibrant personality in a body that doesn't vibrate.

When a body begins to vibrate, the breathing deepens spontaneously and is maintained at a deep level as long as the vibrations continue. The vibrations set the stage for the spontaneous expression of feeling. As the vibrations reach the chest and the larynx, the patient will often begin to sob. I have seen the patient's legs vibrate so strongly that the movement changed spontaneously into kicking. The vibrations also serve to free the pelvis and set it in motion. When the spontaneous pelvic movements become coordinated with the respiratory wave, the orgasm reflex appears, that is, the pelvis swings forward and backward with each breath.

Breathing itself is a self-expressive act which depends on the motility of the organism. Inspiration is an aggressive reaching out to the environment to take in the atmosphere. There is an upward flow of excitation to the head and an active sucking in of air which involves the mouth, pharynx and larynx. During expiration, the excitation flows downward as the air is passively expelled. In a full expiration the wave of excitation can be felt passing down into the genitals or the feet through which it is grounded into the earth. This longitudinal pulsation associated with breathing (the upward flow of excitation during inspiration and the downward flow during expiration) is the basic internal movement from which all self-expressive acts arise.

The upward flow of excitation is concerned with taking in or charging up. All movements which are directed upward, i.e., towards the head, aim to increase the organism's charge. We reach out with our eyes, ears, hands and mouth to take in impressions, substances and affection, all of which stimulate or charge the organism. Movements which are directed downwards are discharging or releasing actions. In this category are such expressive acts as crying, laughing, sex, kicking and running. Normally, the two processes are equal. We can discharge only as much as we have taken in, or charge up only as much as we can discharge. By working with breathing we can raise the level of charge, and therefore, of discharge.

Since the breathing is a total body movement, every action that is fully coordinated with the respiratory wave has an emotional tone. If it is not coordinated with the respiration, it has a mechanical quality. One can say that when the breath of life infuses an action, it endows it with feeling.

In terms of these concepts of energy and pulsation, one can describe four pathological conditions:

1. Low energy: reduced pulsation and feeling
2. Hung-up: the person who is hung up cannot discharge or release his excitation
3. Depressed: the depressed person cannot charge up or increase his level of excitation
4. Anxiety: fear of the internal movements or pulsation.

Self-Expression in Movement

The modalities of conscious expression are physical movement, vocal utterances and the look in the eyes. We can express what we feel through these three channels of communication which correspond roughly to the main channels of sense impression, the skin (touch, taste and smell), the ears and the eyes. In a healthy person the three channels of communication are simultaneously involved in all expression of feeling. If we feel sad, for example, our eyes tear, our voice utters a special crying sound and our body convulses in sobs. Anger is likewise expressed in appropriate movements, sounds and looks. When any one of these channels is blocked the emotion becomes weakened or split.

Bioenergetic therapy employs a number of expressive movements in its aim to restore a patient's motility. These are movements which are commonly suppressed by parents during a child's upbringing. The specific movements we use are kicking, hitting (against the couch), reaching out, sucking, biting, etc. It is surprising how few people can execute these movements gracefully or with feeling. In therapy, these movements are generally combined with various vocal utterances to make them more expressive and to elicit more feeling.

The Voice of the Body

Kicking is a good example of an expressive movement. To kick means to protest. Since a child's right to protest against its parents is generally denied, most people cannot kick with any feeling of conviction or effect. Kicking is a whipping motion in which the whole body participates when the movement is done well. Tension in any part of the body interferes with this whip-like action causing the movement of the legs to be forced and constrained. Continued work with kicking loosens the body, deepens its breathing and integrates its parts. What is true for kicking is equally true for all the other expressive movements. They are expressive when they are total body actions.

There are a number of pathological conditions that seriously disturb the rhythm and coordination of expressive movement. These are:

1. Rigidity: the overall rigidity of a body prevents the flow of excitation and impulse. In a rigid body, the expressive movements become mechanical and are experienced as exercises. The patient feels no pleasure or satisfaction in the movement. Rigid bodies can be (a) hard as steel, (b) wooden, (c) massive like rocks or (d) frozen like ice.

2. Collapsed bodies with poor muscle tone and no integration have considerable difficulty executing expressive movements. Their movements appear as gestures which cannot be sustained or which collapse under stress.

3. Fragmentation: the parts of the body are not unified. Each part moves somewhat independently of the whole. Fragmentation is due to deep, circular tensions which surround the major joints and split the body into segments. These tensions are found at the base of the head, dissociating the head from the body, about the shoulders so that the arms hang like appendages, through the diaphragmatic region splitting the body into seemingly separate halves, in the groin making the legs appear like sticks or pillars, etc.

4. Combinations of rigidity and collapse or rigidity and fragmentation. If a person is to be fully self-expressive, all his chronic muscular tensions must be eliminated. When this is accomplished, the breathing becomes full and free, the energy level of the organism rises and feeling becomes the determinant of behavior. The person who is self-expressive has clear, shining or sparkling eyes, a rich, melodious voice and graceful, easy movements.

LECTURE II: THE EYES AND FEELING

The Expressive Quality of the Eyes

In the first lecture I mentioned that the eyes are an important modality of self-expression. This is because the eyes are intimately and directly connected with feelings.

While the expressive quality of the eyes cannot be fully dissociated from the circumocular region, the expression ones sees in the eyes is determined mainly by changes in the eye itself. To read this expression one should look softly at the eyes of a person, neither fixedly nor staring, until one gets an impression. Almost every feeling that a person is capable of experiencing can be expressed through the eyes. Among the feelings I have seen expressed in people's eyes are the following:

1. Appealing—"Please love me"
2. Longing—"I want to love you"
3. Watchful—"What are you going to do?"
4. Distrustful—"I can't open to you"
5. Erotic—"I am excited by you"
6. Hateful—"I hate you."

The eyes are said to be the mirrors of the soul. This soulful quality is particularly evident in the eyes of a dog or of a cow. Their soft brown eyes are like limpid pools when these animals are relaxed. Each kind of animal has a special look which reflects the quality of the animal. Cats' eyes, for example, have a quality of independence and distance which is very difficult to describe. The eyes of a bird are different, again. Yet the eyes of animals are capable of expressing feeling. After one has lived with a cat or a bird for some length of time, one becomes capable of distinguishing different expressions. I believe that the richness of an organism's inner life is reflected in the range of feeling visible in the eyes.

Because of this expressive quality, the eyes are truly the windows of the body. Thus eyes can be shuttered or open. In the first case they are impenetrable, in the second, one can see into the person. They can be vacant or distant. Vacant eyes give the impression that no one is home. Looking into such eyes one gets a feeling of inner emptiness. Distant eyes indicate that the individual is far away. One can sense his return when the eyes become focused upon one and feeling is expressed. The eyes light up when a person is excited. They dull off when the inner excitation fades out. If the eyes are conceived of as windows, the light that shows in them emanates from the interior of the body. We speak of burning eyes in the face of a zealot who is consumed by some inner fire. There are laughing eyes, sparkling eyes and twinkling eyes. I have actually seen stars in a person's eyes. But there are also sad eyes, which is much more common.

I had an experience once with eyes that I shall never forget. Many years ago my wife and I looked at the eyes of a woman who was sitting opposite us in a subway car. The contact with her eyes gave me a feeling of shock. Her eyes looked so evil that I almost shuddered with horror. My wife had an identical reaction and as we discussed it afterwards, we both agreed that we had never seen such evil-looking eyes. Prior to that experience I don't believe we thought it possible for eyes to look so evil. The incident evoked in my mind stories I had heard about the "evil eye" that has strange and frightening powers. I have subsequently seen another person whose eyes could be described as evil. Both Dr. Pierrakos and I had the same impression from this person's eyes.

The physiological processes that determine the expression of feeling in eyes are largely unknown. We are acquainted with the fact that the pupils narrow in pleasure and widen in states of pain or fear. The narrowing of the pupil increases the focus. Widening the pupil enlarges the field of peripheral vision while reducing the sharpness of focus. These reactions are mediated by the autonomic nervous system but they do not explain the subtle phenomena described above.

The Role of the Eyes in Contact

The eyes actually have a double function: they are organs of vision and also organs of contact. When one's eyes meet those of another person, one actually gets a sensation of physical contact. The quality of this contact varies with the look in the eyes. The look can be so hard and strong that it feels like a slap in the face or so soft that it feels like a caress. Or the look can be penetrating. One can look into a person, through him, over him or around him. If the eyes make contact with the object or person, one can speak of looking as opposed to seeing. Many people see without looking. Looking is an active or aggressive function that embraces but is more than the function of seeing. There is a further discussion of the difference between these two functions in *The Betrayal of the Body*.

Eye contact is one of the strongest and most intimate forms of contact between two people. It is as if the feeling or inner essence of one person touches the feeling or inner essence of another. It is, therefore, a very exciting form of contact. When the eyes of a man and woman meet, the feeling can be so strong that it runs through the body to the pit of the belly and the genitals. The look in such cases is extremely erotic, that is, it is open and inviting. Whatever feeling is involved when eyes meet, the effect of the meeting of eyes is the passing of understanding between the two people.

Eye contact is especially important and significant in the relation between parents and children. It is important because without this contact the young child feels cut off from the parent. It is significant because the looks that pass between parent and child profoundly influence the child's feelings. The look can be loving, affectionate, accepting, rejecting, angry, hateful, contemptuous, derisive, seductive, etc. The father who looks at his young daughter with an erotic expression in his eyes stimulates her sexuality and creates an incestuous bond between them.

The expression of feeling in the eyes can be understood only in terms of the energy pulsation between the head and tail ends of the body. This pulsation is a stream of energy or feeling that extends upward and downward from its center in the region of the solar plexus. At its furthest it reaches and extends upward through the eyes above and downward into and through the genital and legs below. The term energy is used as synonymous with excitation. Thus when the excitation charges the eyes and they light up with feeling, the legs and feet are equally charged and the person feels their contact with the ground. This effect can also be produced in reverse. When the legs become charged with feeling as a result of the various therapeutic exercises, the eyes become brighter. Several patients have commented that after working strongly with their legs, their vision improved to the extent that objects in the room seemed clearer and brighter.

The degree of energy charge in the eyes is a measure of the strength of the ego, one that I use constantly in my practice. The individual with a strong ego has the ability to direct the look in his eyes at another person. Looking at another person is a form of self-assertion just as looking itself is a form of self-expression. When the energy charge in the eyes is strong, they shine or glow. In such persons it can be assumed that the sexual charge is equally strong. These people are sometimes described as "bright-eyed and bushy-tailed."

Many people have difficulty in directing their look due to a weakness in their ability to focus their eyes. This results in a loss of eye contact. With some effort they can bring their eyes into focus to meet another person's look, but I have observed that when they do this, they become embarrassed and avert their gaze. They seem unable to stand the excitation that develops in their bodies. Animals, on the other hand, seem to have the ability to look into a person's eyes unflinchingly, although it is common knowledge that animals become restless when stared at for a continued time.

Eye Disturbances

The eye can be disturbed in either or both of its functions, looking and seeing. The common disturbances of vision are myopia and astigmatism. The disturbances of looking are due to difficulties of focusing and to a lack of strong feeling which would spark the eyes. Generally, the two sets of disturbances coexist. For example, the person who suffers from myopia also has trouble in making eye contact and in expressing feeling through his eyes. I believe that the emotional disturbance is primary in this condition and that the visual disturbance develops secondarily as a result of strain.

In the genesis of eye problems three sets of factors must be considered: heredity, constitution, and environment. There is no proof that heredity plays a part in the origin of myopia although this condition tends to run in families. Children of parents who are myopic are more likely to develop this condition than children of non-myopic parents. The constitutional factor seems important because the ability to focus or to express feeling with the eyes depends on the energy level of the organism. Not all children are born with the same energy level. Weaker infants are characterized by lower weight, poorer respiration, weaker cries, and less aggressive sucking movements. It also takes them a longer time before their eyes become strong enough to focus spontaneously.

The infant's relation to the mother and especially the quality of the eye contact between infant and mother has a decisive effect upon the development of the child's personality and the functioning of its eyes. If the contact between mother and child is pleasurable and satisfying, the mother will look at the child with eyes that are warm, soft, and expressive of the joy she feels in her child. The child responds to this look with pleasure and its eyes become soft and relaxed in turn. Breast-fed babies are continually looking at their mother's eyes while feeding for this expression of feeling.

If an infant encounters a look of extreme anger, rage or hatred in its mother's eyes, its body will experience a shock, particularly in its eyes. Its eyes will become wide with fear, and it will cry or scream. The crying or screaming releases the body from its state of shock and the eyes return to normal. In many situations, however, the scream is blocked. This happens particularly when the mother's anger or hatred is provoked by the baby's crying or screaming. If the shock is not released or if the mother's hostility is experienced repetitively, the infant's eyes tend to open wide in fear of the mother, anticipating an angry look. Wide eyes enlarge the field of peripheral vision but reduce central vision. The child will then attempt to regain its visual acuity by constricting its eyes forcibly, thus creating a condition of rigidity. This rigidity imposes a strain upon the eyes which cannot be maintained indefinitely.

Myopia commonly sets in between the ages of ten and fourteen and can be attributed, in my opinion, to the changes in personality which occur at this time. The developing sexual maturity of the child acts to broaden the field of interpersonal relations and also that of vision. The old conflicts with the parents are often reactivated during this period. I think that what happens then is a collapse of the rigidity that sustained a sharp vision. The eyes become wide again with fear of a non-specific nature. A new defense against the fear is subsequently erected on a lower level. The muscles at the base of the head and about the jaw become contracted to cut off the flow of feeling into the eyes. This ring of tension is found in almost all cases of myopia. It serves to suppress the feeling of fear so that the child can maintain a seemingly normal function.

The myopic eye is in a partial state of shock. This explains why special eye exercises, the Bates method, for example, are often helpful in reducing the disturbance. The wide-eyed look that is typical of myopia is an expression of fear. Yet the individual does not feel any fear nor is he aware of any connection between his eyes and that emotion. There are many cases, however, where myopia does not develop although the conditions for its occurrence are present. In these cases other parts of the body take up the shock, thus sparing the eyes. If the shock to the person resulting from parental hostility and rejection is more severe, the total body becomes affected. A degree of paralysis develops which limits all self-expression and reduces all feeling. The energy level of the organism is decreased, breathing is severely restricted, and motility is low. This condition prevents the possibility of any effective charge in the eyes and permits them to retain their rigidity. Thus, although the sexual development in this personality is weak, myopia may not develop.

The Bioenergetic Therapy of Eye Disturbance

The bioenergetic therapy of eye disturbances in the expression of feeling is based on the above considerations. As with problems of motility and vocal utterance, the energy level of the organism must be raised by a fuller and deeper respiration. The overall effect of deeper breathing is to increase body sensation and feeling. It then becomes imperative to open up the areas of self-expression.

In all cases a considerable amount of work must be done to release the muscular tensions about the jaw and at the base of the head. Releasing the jaw tensions allows feelings to flow up through the throat in vocal utterances. Not infrequently, the patient starts with shouting which then develops into sobbing. The feeling of sadness as expressed in crying and sobbing softens the body and opens the way for the expression of other feelings. Crying has an immediate effect upon the eyes. They become soft and alive. Sometimes they even shine. Patients are often surprised how well their eyes look afterthey have given in to their sadness and cried.

Breathing itself has a direct effect upon the eyes. After sustained deep breathing through the procedures of bioenergetic therapy, the eyes of a person are noticeably brighter. It is immediately evident to the observer. Many patients have commented that they can see better and that the room looks brighter after a session.

The main therapeutic task, however, is to release the blocked fear in the eyes of a patient. The maneuver I use to accomplish this is as follows: I ask the patient who is lying on the bed to hold his open hands about eight inches above his face. He is then directed to open his eyes as wide as possible and to drop his jaw. In this position, the patient assumes an expression of fright. Few, if any, patients feel afraid because the feeling of fear has been blocked. I then ask the patient to look directly into my eyes which are about a foot above his own and I press down firmly with my thumbs on both sides of his nose. This pressure further opens the eyes and prevents the patient from smiling. It removes the mask from the patient's face. If the procedure is done correctly, it will often elicit a scream of fear as the fear wells up in the patient's eyes. When the scream subsides, I remove the pressure, and while the patient is still looking into my eyes, his own become relaxed, their color deepens, tears well up and understanding passes between us.

The procedure doesn't work in every case. Many patients are too frightened to allow the fear to come through. Sooner or later, however, I can elicit the fear. When I do, the effect is remarkable. One patient told me the other day that as she screamed, she saw the eyes of her father looking at her angrily as he was about to beat her. Another told me that he saw the furious eyes of his mother in a recollection that went back to the time he was one year old. One man who had been in therapy for some time was so shook by the experience of his terror that he left my office in a state of collapse like a limp rag. He immediately went home and slept for two hours. He called me shortly after he awoke to say that he had such a feeling of joy at being alive as he had never known before. The joy was a rebound from the release of the terror.

I shall relate one other incident. I saw one young man recently who was cross-eyed. He saw only with one eye, the left one. The vision of the right eye, though normal, was suppressed to avoid a double image. As a child he had had two operations to correct the condition but to no avail. Not only was the right eye turned inward but the right side of his face was slightly twisted. Palpation in the back of the neck revealed a severe muscle spasm on the right side of the nuchal region. I maintained a firm pressure upon this spasm for about thirty seconds and I could feel it let go. Several doctors were watching this young man as he lay on the bed. They were amazed to notice that his eyes became straight and the young man reported that he had single vision with both eyes. The change was dramatic but unfortunately it did not last. The spasm returned later and the eye went off again.

I have not been able to eliminate the myopic condition in any patient's eyes. Much more work would have to be done with the eyes, a la the Bates method, for example, to achieve this result. Many patients tell me that their vision was improved as a result of therapy. This is particularly true for younger patients. In all cases, however, it is possible to restore a greater measure of expressiveness to a patient's eyes. Their eyes can show more feeling and they are able to make better contact with the eyes of another person. I can generally follow a patient's progress by watching this development.

The degree of emotional health can be measured by the amount and range of feeling the eyes can express. Certainly no one can be considered emotionally healthy who cannot make or sustain a feeling eye contact with another person.

5

Thinking and Feeling
The Bioenergetic Analysis of Thought

LECTURE I: THE NATURE OF THOUGHT

Introduction

Thinking is ordinarily regarded as being opposed to feeling. The thinking person is contrasted with the impulsive person, the individual who acts on his feelings without thinking. Stop to think is the command of reason. This antithesis between thinking and feeling is reflected in the dialectic which views these functions as opposing aspects of consciousness and perception. Every movement of the body that is perceived gives rise to both a feeling and a thought. A feeling is perceived against the background of the emotional spectrum and is interpreted on one level as pleasurable or painful, and, on another level, as anger, fear, affection, hostility or a combination of these. A thought arises when a movement is perceived and interpreted in terms of the mental images, visual, auditory, symbolic, etc., that are stored in the brain. The following diagram illustrates this dialectic view.

That body movements give rise to feelings and thoughts is not self-evident. The assumption rests on the fact that dead men have neither feelings nor thoughts. It is supported by repeated observations that feelings depend on movement. When I put my hat on my head I feel it. However, if it remains in the same position for some time I become unconscious of its presence. Should it move, I immediately become aware of it again. If a person doesn't move his arm for a long period, it becomes numb and he doesn't feel it. The reactivation of the circulation through movement restores the feeling. The relation of thought to movement is more complex.

I shall attempt to show that thinking is directly related to feeling and that the antithesis between them is apparent only when their function is viewed from the top of the pyramid, that is, from the position of the ego. All the functions of the personality form a hierarchy the order of which is determined by the level of consciousness. The base is formed by the

Consciousness - Perception

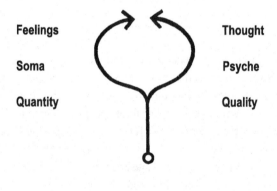

Feelings	Thought
Soma	Psyche
Quantity	Quality

Body Movement

Fig. 1

rhythmic activities of the body which are below consciousness. The first level of consciousness is the perception of pleasure and pain. As consciousness develops, these feelings are elaborated and discriminated into the various emotions. Emotions give rise to thoughts by being transformed into images. In man they undergo a further abstraction into words. A higher level of consciousness permits the development of objective thought and reasoning. At the apex of the pyramid is the ego, the self-conscious self that directs most of our waking activities. The pyramid is shown below.

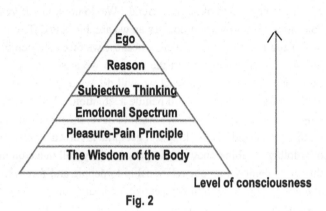

Fig. 2

The Function of Thought

If an animal had no choice of action it would have little need to think consciously. Its reactions would be completely instinctive as in withdrawing from pain or reaching out for pleasure. Such behavior characterizes very young infants and lower forms of life. Most animals, however, are faced with choices that cannot be decided by instinctive behavior alone. A crow approaching food near a house is subject to conflicting feelings. Its hunger draws it to the food but its fear of man holds it back. It moves cautiously, eyes and ears alert, judging the situation and deciding at each moment whether to advance or retreat. A wolf stalking a herd of elk must choose the one it will attack. This choice is partly instinctive and partly based on the evidence of its eyes as to which particular elk is most vulnerable. It must also choose the moment and direction of action.

Our perception of the animal tells us that some form of thinking occurs when conscious choices are made. Confronted with alternative actions the animal may stop and at this moment we sense from its attitude that it may be thinking, not, of course, as humans do. It lacks the ability to frame the possibilities of action in verbal images or other symbolic representations but this ability may be only a higher form of thought and not the essence of thinking in general. We do not know if an animal is conscious of its thought processes as we are, but this difference may be one of degree not of kind. We think because we face innumerable choices in our daily activities. From the moment we arise to the moment we fall asleep we think about what we will do, what clothes we will wear, what we will eat, how we will handle a situation, what we will say, etc. Obviously the more choices we seem to have, the more thinking we are required to do and our thinking can get quite involved. Even in choosing our clothes we think about the impression they will make on others and this often conjures up our relationship to people and forces us to think about them. In our thinking we evoke the images of our complex world, past, present and future, as we try to arrive at the attitudes and actions that will promote our well-being.

The variety of choices may easily lead to a sense of frustration. We feel this frustration keenly when we pick up a piece of jigsaw puzzle and cannot fit it into the picture. On the other hand, we experience a sense of satisfaction when a piece falls neatly into place in the scheme of the puzzle. The frustration and the feeling of satisfaction are physical as well as mental. Frustration represents a block in the flow of feeling through the body, creating a tension that may verge on pain. Fitting the pieces together establishes a connection between the impulse and the picture puzzle that allows the excitation to flow through the body into the world. This outward flow of feeling is, as we saw in the preceding series of lectures, the energetic basis for the experience of pleasure.

Thinking may be defined as the process of making connections between our feelings and the picture we have in our minds of our environment. When a feeling connects or fits perfectly, as in the jigsaw puzzle, we experience a sense of harmony with the environment that is pleasurable. Each feeling that doesn't fit creates tension, pain and frustration. The simpler our lives are, the more easily is this harmony achieved. In a complex society the fit is rarely perfect.

The living process is vastly more complicated than a jig-saw puzzle in which the picture is static and the pieces are immutable. The human environment is constantly changing and our feelings are never the same from one time to another. Each mood and every feeling modifies the structure and form of our being, necessitating new adaptations and requiring us to establish new connections. We are forced to think almost constantly as we endeavor to relate ourselves to the world about us and to formulate the actions that will fulfill our needs.

For the purpose of this discussion, thinking can be divided into three levels: unconscious thinking, conscious thinking and self-conscious thinking. In unconscious thinking the connections are made below the level of awareness. Psychoanalysis has shown that unconscious thoughts dictate behavior often as much as does our conscious thinking. There is considerable evidence that some of our most creative thinking occurs on this level, rising to consciousness later as intuition or inspiration. Arthur Koestler, in *The Creative Act*, describes this process as an unconscious connection between two previously unrelated experiences. This connection may involve such strong charges of excitement that it produces a flash of illumination which Koestler calls the "Eureka reaction."

In conscious thinking the connection is made between an immediate feeling and the environment as directly perceived. In such thinking I connect my feeling of hunger to a suitable source of food, or my feeling of anger to a special situation or an insulting remark. Conscious thinking may also be called subjective thinking.

Self-conscious thinking or objective thinking occurs when the person detaches himself from a feeling or emotion and pictures it in his mind as an image. In the remark, "When I am insulted, I get angry," the connection is made between two images seen from above or without. In such thinking one is aware of one's self and, therefore, of one's thinking. It can also be said that being aware of one's thinking, one is conscious of the self. Descartes took this position in his dictum, "I think therefore I am." I shall analyze this form of thinking more fully later. Human beings have the ability to observe their own thought processes through a superordinate eye, the intellect. This ability gives rise to the consciousness of conscious thinking or self-conscious thinking.

The Role of Deception in Thinking

An interesting aspect of the nature of self-consciousness was revealed by the remarks of one of my patients. She said that she recalled the moment when she became consciously aware of herself. Her parents had demanded an explanation from her for some action and the thought flashed through her mind that she didn't have to answer truthfully. At that moment, she remarked, "I became aware of myself as an independent agent."

Many children go through an early phase of development in which they tell lies. The lie may be a denial of some action which the parents regard as a wrong. A child takes some money that is lying around and hides it. When confronted by his parents with their conviction that he took the money, the child, in the most innocent manner, denies any knowledge of the event. Some time later he may admit his action or the money may be discovered among his possessions. His parents may make a terrible scene and punish the child for lying or if they are wise, they will regard the incident as the child's exploration of deceit and trust that he will learn when to use it properly.

It is interesting to speculate on the relationship between deceit and self-awareness. Consciousness arises, as Erich Neumann shows, from the recognition of differences. To be conscious of light one must know dark, of up one must know down, of you one must know me. Self-consciousness would similarly demand a pair of alternatives. If one can only speak the truth, one lacks a choice and without the choice, consciousness of one's behavior is reduced and control is limited. The recognition that one has a choice strengthens the ego's mastery over the organism's response and, in effect, places the ego in the driver's seat. The ego becomes the center of self-consciousness through its ability to discriminate between truth and falsehood, right and wrong. Can one gain this ability without exploring the realm of deceit?

We should not be disturbed at this idea of a natural role for deceit. In important areas of life it has a positive value. In the game of football, for example, we greatly admire the player who knows how to use deceit to throw his opponent off guard and gain the advantage. The same thing is true of the art of boxing and the strategy of warfare. The ability to mask one's moves and deceive the opponent is often critical to success. The smoothness of a feint which misleads an opponent is the mark of a master not only in the realm of physical combat but in all situations of opposition. In the game of chess or cards, the proper use of deceit may be the difference between victory and defeat. The hunter, whether human or animal, is stealthy. In all such situations, the ability to use deceit is an important asset. It has an obvious negative value in situations which call for cooperation and understanding. It is disastrous if it becomes self-deceit.

To be consciously deceitful in situations of contention requires objectivity. One has to place oneself in the position of the opponent to correctly evaluate the deception. "If I make this move, what will he think?" The success of the deception depends on how accurately one has grasped an opponent's response. Deceit requires that a person step outside of the self and become conscious of the self and the other.

Without the recognition of the existence of deceit, one would never have to take an objective view. A person would respond to the external appearance of a situation without allowing for the possibility that he could deceive or be deceived. He would trust his senses implicitly. Once one recognizes the possibility that our sense impressions may not reveal the full truth of a situation, we must have recourse to the higher faculty of objective thinking or reasoning to insure our security. A human being consciously subjects the evidence of his senses to critical evaluation in the light of past experience stored as knowledge in his mind.

No sense impression will tell us, for example, that iron could be smelted from iron ore. The discovery of iron grew out of the knowledge gained in the course of a bronze culture. It can be said that knowledge, once achieved, sharpens and extends the senses. It arises in the beginning, however, from the recognition that there is another reality behind the surface manifestation.

All animals think to some degree but only human beings know or think objectively. This form of thinking that produces knowledge is a function of the intellect, that aspect of man's mind that enables him to project and evaluate his own thinking and behavior. Each increase in knowledge expands the intellect and forces man into a more objective position. In making him conscious of his own subjectivity and distrustful of it, too, it enhances his individuality and augments his isolation. Because he knows and does not merely trust his senses, man is a conscious actor in the drama of life.

Subjectivity and Objectivity

We think subjectively when our point of reference is within ourselves and our thinking is oriented towards the expression of our feelings and the satisfaction of our desires. To think objectively, the point of reference must be outside the self and the understanding of causal relationships must not be influenced by personal feelings and desires. Objective thinking seeks to define causal relationships in terms of actions rather than feelings. To be objective, thinking must be detached from feeling.

The question arises, can thinking ever be completely divorced from feeling? In fact, when one ponders the nature of objective thought, that is, unemotional thinking, it seems more of a contradiction than subjective thought. If the detachment is complete, the mind divorced from its connection with the sentient aspects of being becomes transformed into a computer that operates only on the basis of information fed into it. This is programmed thinking. In limited situations the human mind can function in this way. The thinking of a student doing a geometry problem resembles the operation of a computer. The student attempts to bring all the information he learned about geometry to the solution of the problem at hand. If this information is incomplete, he cannot solve the problem since neither his feelings nor his personal experience is of much help.

As long as the body of a person is alive it will send impulses to the brain informing that organ of its sensations and feelings and giving rise to subjective thoughts. In the midst of the most abstract deliberations one is not free from the intrusion of personal consideration, feelings of irritation, frustration, pleasure, pain, etc. These intrusions make the task of objective thinking difficult and it often requires a considerable effort of will to remain objective under these conditions. The intrusions will be minimal when the body is in a state of pleasure and the objective thinking will reflect the positive tone of the body. Painful feelings represent a greater disturbance since pain is always interpreted as a danger signal. To think objectively when the body is in a state of pain (lack of pleasure) one has to deaden the body. Such a "deadening" dissociates the mind from the body and makes the quality of the thinking mechanical or computerized. Creative thinking, which depends on the free flow of unconscious ideas, occurs only when the body is most alive and unburdened. The quality of one's thinking and probably the content, too, can never be fully divorced from the emotional tone of the body.

Objective thinking becomes most difficult when a person attempts to be objective about his own behavior. Since behavior is largely determined by feelings, a person has to be cognizant of his feelings to evaluate his behavior objectively. For example, if a person is unaware of his hostility, he will explain the negative reactions he meets by other people's ill feelings. He cannot, of course, see his actions as others see them and he will be unable to assess his role in provoking a negative response. Unaware of his hidden emotions and motives, he cannot be fully objective about himself. The eye of the intellect can only evaluate the logic of one's reasoning. On the other hand, if a person is conscious of his feelings and can express them subjectively, he can take an objective position: he can say, for example, "I realize that I am hostile and I can see why people are reacting negatively to me." True objectivity requires a proper subjectivity.

Thinking can never be divorced from feeling. Since everything a person does is determined by his desire for pleasure and his fear of pain, no act can be entirely unbiased, no action can be without some personal interest. It follows logically that every thought is related to a feeling and will either support the feeling or oppose it according to the characterological attitude of the individual. One can reach the same conclusion from the dialectical analysis of the relation between thinking and feeling since both the thought and the feeling arise from the perception of a body movement.

To be truly objective one must recognize and declare one's personal attitude or feeling. Without this subjective basis the attempt to be objective ends in a pseudo-objectivity. The psychological term that characterizes such pseudo-objectivity is rationalization. The mechanism of rationalization is to deny the subjective feeling that motivates a thought or an action and to justify one's behavior by causal reasoning. "You made me do it." Rationalization is an attempt to place the responsibility for one's actions on the other person or outside situation. Will Durant remarks, "Reason, as every school girl now informs us, may be only the technique of rationalizing desire."

Objective thought offers little help in the multitude of problems and conflicts that arise daily in our lives. No mother could respond to her child on the basis of objective thought. If she interprets her baby's cry correctly, it will not be on the basis of logic but because she senses through empathy the feeling behind the cry and responds with feeling to the baby's need. In all interpersonal relationships, how we behave and what we say is controlled by subjective thinking. One cannot relate to another person objectively because an objective relationship reduces individuals to objects.

The problem of thinking is that people cannot think objectively because they do not think subjectively. All great philosophic thinking contains a strong subjective bias which is apparent to a sensitive reader and which adds flavor to the writing. People do not think subjectively because they have been taught (1) to regard such thinking as inferior, (2) to distrust their feelings and justify their actions by reasons, and (3) that pleasure is never a sufficient aim in life. The result is that they have lost touch with their feelings.

Thinking starts with feeling and leads to wisdom. Obviously, since not all thinking leads to wisdom, I would ascribe the fault to the lack of a genuine feeling. To know thyself is the essence of wisdom.

LECTURE II: NEGATION AND THINKING

Knowledge and Self-Assertion

I have postulated the hypothesis that the growth of consciousness proceeds from the basic pleasure-pain sensations through the spectrum of emotions to thinking. The emotional reactions retain an instinctive quality. They are not primarily learned responses even though they depend on a measure of muscular coordination for their expression. Thinking, on the other hand, cannot be dissociated from learning and the acquisition of knowledge. When consciousness develops to the point where thought is possible, learning occurs and knowledge results.

The step from impulsive response to thinking requires the introduction of a frustration and a negation. If the instinctive actions of an organism were capable of fulfilling all its needs and desires, conscious thought would be unnecessary. It is only where instinctive patterns of behavior fail to satisfy the organism that the need for thought arises. In all the learning experiments with animals, frustration is the lever that forces the animal to learn a new behavior and achieve a desired end. In one of the most famous of these experiments a banana was placed outside the cage of an ape, just beyond his reach. After a number of unsuccessful attempts to reach the banana with his arm, the ape finally noticed a stick that had been left in its cage. Using the stick as an extension of its arm it was able to retrieve the banana. On subsequent occasions, recourse to the stick occurred after fewer unsuccessful efforts to reach the banana with its hand. It can be said that the ape learned a new skill, that the learning involved thinking and that in the process it acquired the knowledge of how to use the stick in a new way.

The role of frustration in thinking is obvious, that of the negation is obscure. Frustration does not necessarily lead to thinking; it may just as easily turn into anger and rage. These, in fact, are the more natural responses. Thinking can only happen when the frustrated desire is shunted away from this natural avenue of release. Sometime before the frustration becomes overwhelming, the organism must stop the impossible effort. Stop to think, as I pointed out in the first lecture, is an old maxim. The "stop" that is so essential to thinking is an unspoken "No," a negative command from a higher center that holds back the instinctive reaction.

We often hear that people in a moment of danger use the same method to save themselves. I recently heard about a young man who was caught in a dangerous undertow and found that he could not extricate himself from it despite his best efforts to swim. Realizing that he was becoming frightened and desperate, he said to himself, "Don't panic." A moment's thought told him that he should save his strength and call for help. He did this and was rescued.

Let us now pursue this question a little differently. As an infant grows older it will inevitably come into conflict with its parents. But let us assume that it has an unusual nature, that it listens to everything its mother says and follows her command to the letter. "Eat this puree," the mother commands and the child obeys faithfully. If this program were continued, how would the child ever learn to think? It would have no need to think since mother knows best. It would have no need to learn since mother would foresee all problems and handle all contingencies. It would gain no knowledge since it would have no need of knowledge. Fortunately, no child is born naturally with such a disposition, for it would become a helpless idiot.

When a child obeys a command it is deprived of an opportunity to think, to learn and to acquire knowledge. This is not to say that one must never command a child. Commands are necessary in emergencies but not in learning situations. The latter requires a free play of wills if thinking is to occur.

Most children go through a negative phase in the course of their growth and development. Between eighteen months and two years of age they will frequently say "No" to parental demands and offerings. This "No" expresses the child's desire for independence and its right to make its own choices. It is often so spontaneous that the child may say "No" to something it wants. I recall offering my young son a cookie he liked. Before he even recognized it, he turned his head away in a gesture of rejection. A second look convinced him it was a desired object and he reached for it. In our dealings with people it is much easier to change a "No" to "Yes" than a "Yes" to "No." The "Yes" is a commitment which binds two parties; the "No" leaves them free for further exchanges.

Whether we permit a child to make its own choice in any situation depends on the circumstances of that situation. In principle we must always respect a child's right to say "No." If this right is denied, the child will react with anger and hostility that will grow in proportion as its ability to stand up to and oppose its parents is frustrated. When the early efforts of a child to establish a self-regulatory pattern and to assert its individuality are rebuffed by the parents, a situation of conflict will develop that will be most difficult to overcome later.

The imposition of patterns of response is popularly called brain-washing. To brain-wash a person, his resistance and will must be overcome. He must, in effect, be deprived of the right to say "No." As long as he has that right, he will attempt to find things out for himself. When patients are incapable of voicing their opposition they are likewise incapable of finding out anything for themselves. They look to the therapist for answers that he doesn't have. When one asks them a question they answer, "I don't know." They cannot think, they do not learn and they have no knowledge of life. Fortunately, very few patients are completely brain-washed. Most patients suffer from a relative limitation of their ability to assert their opposition, but it is this limitation that is responsible for their problems and their lack of knowledge.

Negation and Individuality

Every organism is surrounded by a membrane that separates it from its environment and determines its individuality. This limiting membrane of the body is the organ of sensation (sensing). An organism will feel (react to) whatever impinges on its surface from without or acts on the surface from within. Without a limiting membrane a movement will not give rise to sensation or feeling. A free wave such as occurs in a body of water creates no sensation in the water. The same wave in an organism can cause a feeling when the inner movement reaches the limiting membrane or surface of the body.

In *Physical Dynamics of Character Structure* I discussed the function of perception in relation to the internal events of the body. Many events or movements occur within the body which do not reach consciousness. We are not ordinarily aware of the heart's activity, we do not perceive the intestinal movements, and we do not sense the production and internal flow of urine. Sensation arises and perception occurs only when an internal activity affects the surface of the body. For example, when the heart beats with such force that it causes a thumping of the chest one becomes aware of the sensation of the heart pounding. Theoretically, impulses arise at the center of an organism and are directed towards objects in the external world. However, we are not conscious of our impulses until they reach the surface where an action can take place which will satisfy the aim of the impulse. Thus, one cannot perceive an impulse that fails to reach the surface of the body.

Perception also involves the mind, specifically the surface of the mind where consciousness is believed to be located. Anatomically, consciousness is related to the cortex of the cerebral hemispheres. Two phenomena combine to form a perception: (1) an impulse reaches the surface of the body; (2) a message reaches the surface of the brain. The two events occur almost simultaneously and it is as if the events which occur at the surface of the body are projected upon the surface of the mind. In many respects, the mind is like a mirror which reflects in consciousness what is taking place on the body's surface in actuality. And just like a mirror cannot show what goes on beneath the surface, so too is consciousness limited to surface phenomena. Freud had described the ego as a projection of a surface upon a surface. The ego embraces the functions of perception and consciousness. In *Physical Dynamics of Character Structure* I stated: "Experiments have confirmed the fact that sensation occurs when an internal movement reaches the surface of the body and of the mind where the system perception-consciousness is located." The interested reader is referred to this book for a more detailed analysis of these functions.

In the human organism the limiting membrane of the body is composed of the skin and the underlying layers of striated or voluntary muscles. A membrane that is too flexible or lacks cohesion will allow impulses to pass through without adequate ego control and before these impulses have been fully registered in consciousness. The behavior of such persons will be either impulsive or hysterical. And despite considerable movement, hyperactivity or violent outbursts, feeling is actually reduced. These people show a deficiency of self-containment or self-possession and their egos will be described as weak. They do not know why they behave as they do. An inflexible membrane due to muscular rigidity decreases an individual's expression of impulses and also reduces feeling. In the rigid person there is an absence of spontaneity and behavior tends to be compulsive and mechanical.

The limiting membrane also serves a protective function with regard to incoming stimuli. It allows the individual to screen and distinguish stimuli and prevents the personality from being overwhelmed by such stimuli. For this function, too, the quality of the membrane is important. A thin-skinned person, for example, is hypersensitive; a thick-skinned individual is insensitive. Without a skin a person would be so sensitive that any force acting on his body would be extremely painful.

The "No" functions as a psychological membrane that parallels in every way the physiological membrane of the body. It prevents the individual from being overwhelmed by outside pressures and allows him to discriminate among the demands and inducements to which he is constantly subject. It guards against impulsiveness, for the person who can say "No" to others can also say "No" to his own impulses. By saying "No" to one's self, one has time to think and one's behavior loses the frantic or hysterical character it might otherwise have in a crisis. It prevents rigidity, for rigidity is an unexpressed "No."

I have been asked, "What about the person who says "No" but can't say "Yes"? Doesn't a person have to be able to say "Yes"? My argument is that a person cannot make a meaningful assent unless he is able to say "No." In the absence of the ability to say "No," an assent is merely a form of submission and is not the expression of an individual who has a freedom of choice. The person who cannot say "Yes" is afraid of commitment because he is unsure of his own mind. To know your mind is to mind your "No."

"No" is an expression of opposition which is the cornerstone of individuality. The child who opposes his parents is saying, "I am me, I am different, I have a mind of my own." Such a child will learn to think for himself whereas the "good," obedient child sacrifices his individuality and loses his ability to think for himself. When we teach children we want "good," quiet pupils who will repeat what we have taught them. In such an authoritarian educational process, a child learns nothing of significance for he has gained no knowledge that is personally meaningful. If a child is to learn, he must be given the right to say "No," to oppose his teacher, and to assert his personal ideas and preferences.

The applicability of this principle was tested by one of my patients who taught a first grade class in the public schools of New York. Most of her pupils came from disadvantaged homes and a number had emotional difficulties that interfered with the class routine. One of the constant problems in the class was a restlessness which often disrupted her program. In the middle of each morning and afternoon session, this teacher had her pupils form a line and march about the classroom stamping their feet and shouting, "No! I won't! No! I won't!" This procedure was followed by some breathing exercises. No attempt was made to evaluate the results of this practice objectively but my patient told me how surprised she was to see the calming effect this practice produced in her pupils. They were much more receptive to her and to the school work following the expression of their negativity.

The restlessness of these pupils can be traced to the tensions that result from suppressed negativity. Since the "No" cannot be eliminated it becomes structured in chronic muscular tensions. The unexpressed "No" becomes a ring of contraction about the base of the head, immobilizing that member in a stubborn, unyielding attitude. One finds that the muscles of the nuchal region and the scalenes are tense and contracted. These tensions inhibit the free movement of the head. The jaw is often set in a rigid defiant pose with extremely tight jaw muscles. There are restrictions in the throat to repress the scream. It can be shown that all chronic muscular tension represents an unconscious negation. The basis for this statement is the knowledge that every chronically contracted muscle decreases motility and reduces feeling. In effect, the body is saying, "I won't move and I won't feel."

The reduction of feeling undermines the subjective quality of thought and distorts its objectivity. Instead of clear thinking the mind is preoccupied with rationalizations of unconscious resistance and justifications for submissiveness and rebellion.

The Critical Faculty

In his delightful series of essays, *Portraits from Memory*, Bertrand Russell makes the following observation about himself, "Always the skeptical intellect, when I have most wished it silent, has whispered doubts to me, has cut me off from the facile enthusiasms of others, and has transported me into a desolate solitude." But can anyone be a creative thinker without such an intellect? Can anyone have a real intellect without a screen of skepticism?

The skepticism of Russell is an expression of his individuality and his independence. It is the attribute of a free thinker who forms his own judgments on the basis of his own experience. No one can doubt Russell's ability to say "No." He was arrested in 1915 for expressing his opposition to Britain's entry into World War I. He was ostracized by his liberal colleagues for opposing Russian communism in the 1920s. He was condemned for organizing opposition to the Vietnam War in 1965. Whatever judgment one may make of his actions, no one can question the courage and integrity that prompted those actions. This courage and integrity cannot be dissociated from the quality of Russell's thinking.

It would be a grave error to believe that Russell lacked enthusiasm. From what I know about the man and from what I read in his writings I would say he is in love with life, positive in his outlook, and constructive in his point of view. His intellectual skepticism is the moderating restraint which a secure ego exercises over an enthusiastic nature. By contrast, the facile enthusiasms of the average individual are a desperate search for meaning and assurance. Lacking an inner core of conviction, the insecure person attaches himself to any principle that will serve for the moment to support his faltering ego. Russell writes with a high degree of objectivity because he is at the same time highly subjective.

Progress in the acquisition of knowledge depends on the questioning and denial of established concepts. No forward move in thinking can be made without transcending and, therefore, changing a previous formulation. Copernicus rejected the Ptolemaic concept of the relation between the heavenly bodies. Darwin denied the scholastic view of the origin of species and Einstein disclaimed the applicability of Newtonian physics to astronomical phenomena. Psychoanalysis would not have uncovered the secrets of the unconscious if Freud had not challenged the accepted ideas of hysteria. These achievements were possible because these men had a mind of their own and the courage to say "No." The inquiring mind is a skeptical intellect in an eager and enthusiastic nature.

The core of individuality is a mind that reflects the unique experiences of the individual. A parallel proposition is that each person has a unique body that expresses the feelings of his unique existence. Every person has something to add to the store of knowledge based on the individuality of his life but his contribution is dependent on the acceptance of his individuality and the recognition of his right to dissent. Deprive him of this right and you destroy his individuality. Suppress this right and you leave him open to being brain-washed.

Brain-washing is not a technique invented by the Chinese communists. Indoctrination occurs in the home, in the school and in the community. It takes place whenever a person is forced to accept a statement as true that conflicts with his feelings. How frequently do mothers override a child's objections with the statement "It's good for you." Once the validity of feeling as a guide to behavior is undermined, a child can be taught anything. He is generally taught that his superiors have all the answers and that he is to look to them for direction. He becomes an "outer-directed" person, marked by facile enthusiasms and influenced by all the popular fashions.

The skeptical intellect recognizes the possibility of deceit, conscious or otherwise. Faced with the possibility of deception, the person with a critical faculty uses his reasoning power to avoid the snare. The brain-washed person, on the other hand, is vulnerable because he refuses to face the possibility of deceit. Having cut off his feelings and repressed his opposition, he is without a leg to stand on. He does not see the hostile intentions in others because he has suppressed his own hostility. He cannot cope with negativity because he has rejected his own "No." The thinking of such a person is superficial and his attitude is naive.

It is naive to assume, for example, that the wicked are punished and the good rewarded. It is naive to believe that love conquers all. The woman who marries a profligate and thinks that through her devotion and self-denial she will reform him is naive. The college professor who proclaims that reason can solve all of mankind's problems, and I know such a professor, is naive. His personal life is a failure. It is naive to think that with enough money we will conquer all diseases, eliminate all poverty, and create a Great Society. The cynic has an answer to such delusions. The rich get richer and the poor get poorer.

Morality has a meaning when a person who is capable of being deceitful chooses to be honest out of self-respect. Thinking gains the stature of reason when a person can relate the objective events of his life to his subjective experiences. Without self-knowledge one is neither moral nor rational. Naiveté is a form of self-deceit.

LECTURE III: TRUTH, BEAUTY AND REASON

Sensing and Knowing

There are two ways of apprehending reality, subjectively and objectively. We learn about reality through our senses and also through information that is passed on to us in the form of knowledge. These two ways may seem in many instances to contradict each other. In our technological culture where knowledge is so important we tend to favor objective reality with the result that we deprecate and even at times deny the validity of subjective reality. Such a choice splits the unity of modern man cutting him off from the roots of his instinctual life and thereby increasing his dependence on objective and "scientific" knowledge.

Much of the reality we confront in our daily lives is of a different order than the reality uncovered by science. Despite scientific proof that the earth is round, our ordinary movements are dictated by sense impressions that tell us the earth is flat. In this instance we can neither dismiss the subjective evidence of our senses nor the objective scientific knowledge. Knowing and sensing, apparently so contradictory here, must nevertheless be integrated by the individual. But perhaps knowing and sensing are not contradictory but complementary aspects of a unitary function such as ego-id or mind-body, neither of which can exist without the other.

Objective truth is the sum of man's knowledge at any time and changes, therefore, as his knowledge increases. There is, then, no absolute objective truth. This concept is dramatically illustrated in our understanding of matter. We thought we knew the nature of matter when Rutherford and Bohr described the atom as made up of a nucleus and concentric rings of electrons. We thought that the atoms were immutable, each atom having its own special nucleus. The story of nuclear physics is the discovery that atoms are transmutable since they are composed of similar particles. The electron is no longer viewed as a particle of matter but a field of electrical charge. We have finally reached the boundary between matter and energy and it is questioned whether matter exists at all.

What validity is there to subjective truth? Sensing is a personal and private action in that it involves the interpretation of stimuli in terms of the individual's experience. Subjective truth is, therefore, not absolute either. It varies with the perceptive acuity and the experience of the individual. To what extent then do our senses convey a true picture of reality to us?

True as opposed to false means that our understanding of a situation enables us to predict the outcome of a course of action. If a scientist correctly calculates the interplay of forces in space flight, he will, theoretically at least, be able to predict that a rocket would land on the moon. When it does, we would say that his calculations were true. Objective truth is capable of objective proof. Subjective truth also has a predictable quality. If I sense a patient's anxiety I can confirm the truth of my observation by inquiring about her condition. A husband sensing the hostility of his wife can predict that a jocular tone will meet with a cold-shoulder response.

Subjective truth cannot be verified by objective demonstration. However, if my patient denies her anxiety or the wife denies that she is hostile, the validity of my impression is questioned but not negated. This validity derives from the genuineness of my feeling or that of the husband.

In the conflict that arises when one's sensed observation is denied by the other person, an individual has no choice but to have faith in his own feeling. To turn against his feeling is to undermine his integrity. He cannot claim that what he senses is true of the other person; he can only state that he truly or genuinely had this sense impression. And he cannot act contrary to his sense impression if he is to act honestly. However, he need not act at all if he is not sure of himself.

Self-confidence stems from self-knowledge. The person who lacks self-confidence doesn't trust himself because he doesn't know himself. He is unaware of his motives, uncertain of his feelings, and out of touch with his needs. All forms of psychotherapy aim at self-realization through self-awareness or self-knowledge.

There are two ways to approach the self. The inner self is directly accessible through sensing and feeling and indirectly accessible through the interpretation of behavior, thoughts, fantasies and dreams. This indirect, analytic or objective way forces the person to get outside the self and to some degree splits the unity of the personality. As a result, the knowledge so gained lacks conviction unless it is confirmed and supported by subjective truth acquired directly by sensing and feeling.

In the first lecture I postulated that a feeling arises through the perception of a movement. Sensing is an extension and elaboration of the function of feeling. The two words are often used interchangeably. One can say, "I sense that you are angry," or "I feel that you are angry." Sensing is generally more subtle than feeling. The actual senses are highly developed and differentiated aspects of feeling. They extend our awareness by making us sensitive to minute changes in the body, changes so subtle that they would not ordinarily give rise to a feeling. The sense of hearing is the ability to perceive the slight vibrations of the ear drum. The sense of sight depends on chemical changes in the retina produced by the energy of light. But seeing also requires some movement of the eye. It is not generally appreciated that an eye that is absolutely immobile soon loses the power to discriminate objects.

The concept that without movement there is neither sensing nor feeling underlies the bioenergetic approach to therapy. By increasing the motility of the body the functions of sensing, feeling and thinking are enhanced. Motility is increased by releasing the chronic muscular tensions that have developed in the course of an upbringing that denied full instinctual gratification to the child. The technique is based on the sequence: movement > sensing-feeling > thinking. The analytic approach reverses the order. Beginning with the thought or fantasy it aims to evoke the feeling and thereby restore the motility of the body.

The bioenergetic approach leads directly to the subjective truth of the self. This statement can be illustrated by the following example.

A patient lying on the bed and kicking with his legs senses that he is restraining the movements. Encouraged to extend himself, he becomes aware that he is afraid to "let go." As he tries to do so, he realizes that his fear of "letting go" stems from suppressed rage and that if he did lose control he could do considerable damage. The self-knowledge gained through the interpretation and analytic approach is objective until it gains subjective validity by arousing feeling and restoring motility. Until it does this, it remains tenuous and must be tested anew in every situation. While a combined approach is the most effective therapeutic procedure, it must be realized that the therapeutic goal is self-knowledge based on subjective truth.

Only the truth of the self, experienced directly in the body, can inspire the confidence that one can rely on one's feelings. And only such confidence can build a self-esteem that will withstand the vicissitudes of life. For contrary to popular belief, success and objective knowledge are unstable foundations for self-esteem. A confidence built on success is vulnerable to the first failure. And a confidence in one's actions based on the data of science or the dictum of authority crumbles when extended research challenges the prevailing view. Do you remember when Watson and the Behaviorists told mothers not to pick up their crying babies?

Confidence based on the truth of one's feelings enables one to apprehend reality directly and immediately. Yet problems may arise when subjective truth seems to conflict with so-called objective knowledge. For example, what is to determine our choice of food? Should our selection be based on pleasure and taste or on a knowledge of dietetics?

Some years ago an experiment was carried out on very young children to test whether their natural tastes and preferences would insure an adequate diet. The children were divided into two groups. One group was permitted to choose its diet from a large variety of food. The diet for the other group was carefully prescribed by several doctors. The health of the two groups of children was studied for a period of years, the growth and vitality of each child being carefully observed and noted. At the end of the experiment the doctors conceded that the children who had followed their natural inclinations in the choice of food had prospered better than those whose diet was scientifically selected.

The children followed their desire for pleasure in their choice of food and it worked well. Obviously they did not know the nutritional value of the food they selected and relied wholly on their sense of sight, smell, touch and taste. The question arises, why doesn't this hold true for adults? Why cannot adults follow their natural inclinations in the choice of food with confidence that their choices are healthful? Specifically, why do so many people have to watch their diet rigorously to avoid becoming overweight?

Overeating is a sign, as many doctors are aware, that the self-regulatory processes of the body have broken down. Self-regulation is governed by the pleasure principle. If a person ate for pleasure, his consumption would be regulated by his need since pleasure results from the satisfaction of a need. The overeater, however, is a compulsive eater for whom food has become charged with secondary meanings. Food can be a status symbol for the gourmet or a soporific for the anxious individual. Eating can express rebellion against or submissiveness to a domineering mother, and food can represent survival or indulgence. Whatever the unconscious reason, compulsive eating is often indiscriminatory and taste plays a minor role in regulating this activity. On the other hand, people for whom food is not charged with secondary meanings in their unconscious minds can eat what they want, enjoy their food and retain their normal weight.

The point I wish to make is that feelings are reliable guides to action. If a person could follow his feelings, his life would provide a maximum of pleasure and a minimum of pain. The trouble is that no adult can follow his feelings unless he was permitted to do so as a child. When the self-regulatory and self-expressive processes of the body are disturbed, guilt arises, anxiety develops and tensions are created. The result is internal conflict, ambivalence, and confusion. One no longer knows what he truly feels or wants. The subjective truth of the body has been lost and the individual turns to objective knowledge as a substitute.

163

Such a situation inexorably leads to a progressive alienation from the self and a further deterioration of hedonistic self-regulation. It can only be overcome by a rediscovery of the self.

Similarly, our sense impressions are valid criteria for judging the truth of the world we inhabit. This validity is not negated by radio waves we do not hear, infrared beams of light we cannot see or poisons that elude our taste. In these special areas knowledge must illuminate the unknown. In a world that grows increasingly complex through technological advances, we are handicapped if we lack the knowledge that enables us to cope with the new conditions of living. If, however, we lose touch with our feelings and lose faith in our sense perceptions, we become vulnerable in another direction. We become naive and assume that anything promoted as new, modern or scientific carries an authority we cannot question. Much of the success of advertising stems from this naiveté of people.

True knowledge extends our senses, it doesn't contradict them. When our senses tell us that a person looks ill, we expect knowledge to inform us about the nature of his ailment. It makes no sense for medical science to describe a person as healthy when his appearance belies that fact. Yet this happens all the time. Few physicians see the vacant eyes, the gaunt look, the constricted bodies of schizoid patients or the tight jaws and inflated chests of neurotics. Perhaps they see these signs but do not trust their sense impressions. The priority given to objective truth distorts reality. For each of us, as sentient beings, the subjective truth of our feelings and sense impressions is the touchstone for our apprehension of reality.

Beauty and Grace

People generally feel that the truth is beautiful. This feeling corresponds to another general feeling that falsehood and dishonesty are ugly. The subject I would like to discuss is the relation of beauty to truth. Is it valid to say that beauty is truth? This is a question I would prefer not to answer in the abstract but with reference to my special field of psychiatry.

Beauty is not generally considered to be within the purview of psychiatry. The idea that beauty is in any way connected to mental health seems an odd thought. Any number of psychiatrists will testify that beautiful women and good-looking men can be found among the insane. I have not found one schizoid patient who felt that her body was beautiful, and I would concur in that self-perception. It would be strange if no relationship existed between the beautiful and the healthy. It may be that our ideas of beauty and health need revision.

Healthy children strike us as beautiful; we admire their bright eyes, clean complexions and shapely bodies. Our appreciation of the animal is based on its vitality, its grace and its exuberance. Conversely, illness or disease has a repelling effect. It is difficult to see beauty in illness. In Samuel Butler's *Erewhon*, illness was the only crime for which people in that utopia were jailed.

Yet it offends our sensibilities to think of a sick person as being ugly. We sympathize with his misfortune, especially if the sick person is close to us, and consequently we disavow any repugnance the illness may evoke in us. Such sentiments are particularly human; the wild animals destroy their sick.

If beauty is divorced from health, it is dissociated from the most meaningful aspect of existence. The Greeks, whose culture forms a cornerstone of our own, did not make a distinction between beauty and health. Physical beauty was admired as an expression of health. Their sculpture shows their reverence for the beauty of the human body.

If beauty and physical health are related, what connection exists between beauty and mental health? This is the same thing as asking what connection exists between mental and physical health.

The dichotomy that exists in medicine between the mental and the physical derives from a mechanistic view of health and illness. In the absence of a demonstrable lesion, physicians are reluctant to describe a disturbance as illness. They are suspicious of malingering and unprepared or unwilling to face the social and ethical questions that a positive view of health would entail. In their effort to avoid subjectivity they ignore their senses and rely upon their instruments. No instrument can gauge the state of function of a living organism. What is healthy is a difficult determination to make but it is one that cannot be avoided if the fragmentation of our way of life is to be overcome.

When we look at a healthy child we do not see its state of health. That is a judgment. What we see is a picture that strikes us as beautiful and we interpret it as a manifestation of health. Similarly, a beautiful animal is assumed to be healthy. What is the basis of this assumption?

We think of beauty as something pleasing to the eyes: a beautiful picture, a beautiful woman, a beautiful landscape. Beauty denotes a harmony of the elements, the absence of manifest disproportions and the presence of an inner excitement that irradiates the total view. But beauty is not limited to the visual sense. Music is beautiful when it is pleasing to our ears. Cacophony or even a discordant sound may make us wince.

The pleasure of the beautiful stems from its ability to excite our bodily rhythms and to stimulate the flow of feeling. Our senses and feelings combine to tell us how we respond. If the rhythm is broken and the flow disturbed, the feeling will be painful. Such a response should tell us that our reaction is negative. The response to the beautiful is direct and immediate and requires no interpretation. When this response is lacking, the person senses no beauty. The appreciation of beauty may demand in some cases the development of a special taste but in all cases it is predicated on the bodily feeling of excitement and flow.

In the animal organism, the excitement and flow of feeling associated with pleasure are manifested physically as grace. Grace is the beauty of motion and complements the beauty of form in a healthy organism. Grace has a connotation that suggests superior personal qualities. It is used as a term of reverence. The salutation "Your Grace" denotes that the person so addressed has a special power, a grace that is derived ultimately from kinship with a deity.

The Bible tells us that man was created in the image of God and, presumably, each man possessed grace, that is, he was God-like. Man fell from grace when he ate the fruit of the tree of knowledge and began to think about right and wrong. He must have felt like the centipede who became paralyzed when he tried to figure out which leg to move first. The moment one thinks about moving, the spontaneous flow of feeling through the body is interrupted, producing a gracelessness.

The person endowed with grace is also gracious. He is open, warm and giving. He gives without effort, for every movement of his body is a pleasure to himself and others. He is warm because no tensions limit his breathing and restrict the flow of his energy. He is open because he has not developed any neurotic or schizoid defenses against life.

In a human being the lack of grace is due to chronic muscular tensions that interfere with the rhythmic movements of his body. Each tension pattern represents a conflict that was resolved by the inhibition of certain impulses. If the lack of grace is caused by repressed emotional conflicts, the presence of grace is a sign of emotional health. And if beauty of movement is a mark of emotional health, then beauty of form should have the same meaning.

Since the beautiful is pleasurable, its connection with mental health is clear. The individual capable of taking and giving pleasure, that is, the individual capable of fully experiencing pleasure is emotionally healthy. Such a person is a beautiful individual since his features and expression radiate his good feelings. His eyes aren't empty, his lips aren't tight, his jaw is not grim, his body isn't frozen and his smile isn't fixed. His eyes are bright, his lips are full and parted, his jaw is relaxed, his body is soft yet firm, and his smile is warm and spontaneous. His features show a degree of harmony that reflects the integration of his personality. Such a person is not only emotionally healthy; he is physically healthy in the true sense of health.

A sense of beauty and grace is innate in people. Many persons would admit, I believe, that the current values in feminine pulchritude contradict their inner sense of beauty. When a child sees a truly beautiful woman, it remarks spontaneously, "You're beautiful." Too many people, however, are like the crowd in the story of "The Emperor's Clothes" who have been brain-washed into accepting the dictates of fashion for the subjective truth of their senses. People who are slaves to fashion have surrendered their personal taste in exchange for conformity.

Beauty and grace are the goals to which our conscious efforts are directed. We want to be more beautiful and more graceful because we sense that it is the way to more joy. Beauty is the subject of much of our thinking, the beauty of our personal appearance, the beauty of our surroundings, and the beauty of our work. Beauty and grace are the truth of our being. Despite this fact, the world grows uglier all the time. Has beauty become an adornment rather than a virtue? Something is gravely amiss in our thinking. We have divorced reason from beauty.

Reason and Instinct

Reasoning, like beauty, provides pleasure. In fact, we often describe a particularly fine thought or analysis as beautiful. In the course of my own work I have had many occasions when a seemingly correct interpretation of a problem produced a wave of excitation that I experienced as pleasurable. This pleasure was physical, a heightened rhythmic activity in my body that was so strong it made me get up and move. Intellectual pleasure partakes of the general nature of pleasure, and it is a form of snobbery to consider one pleasure superior to another.

We reason because we are dissatisfied. There is disorder in our personal world, and through our reasoning we attempt to set it right in our minds. This disorder may be due to an unsolved crossword puzzle, a motor that won't start, a child that isn't happy or a theory that doesn't explain our feelings. Whatever the cause of the disorder, it is one that escapes our immediate comprehension and forces us to survey the situation from a different vantage point.

Reasoning is a form of objective thinking in which a problem is viewed from different positions that suggest alternate possibilities. When one of these fits and establishes a connection we feel a degree of satisfaction in our progress towards order. Each step in a reasoning process changes the point of reference and opens new possibilities of understanding. If a problem is circumscribed we can sometimes reason it out. In the larger affairs of life, however, our reasoning only arrives at approximations that leave the picture still incomplete.

Unlike the other animals that live in a natural state of harmony with their world, man, the knowing animal, can experience this harmony only briefly. By his education and culture he becomes an individual and all his conscious energy aims at the assertion of his individuality. The more he knows, the broader is his consciousness and the more separated will he feel from the totality of nature. By his origin and in his unconscious, he senses that he is part of the whole and his bodily effort is directed towards reestablishing the connection. At the height of the sexual orgasm he experiences the joy of reunion but when it is over he awakens to the reality that he has been expelled from the Garden of Eden. This conflict between his conscious individuality and his unconscious identity with the cosmos, between knowing and feeling, forces him to reason. Through his reasoning he develops a personal philosophy.

Every true individual is a philosopher in his own right. He is a lover of wisdom, a seeker of truth, a man who has an "integrated and consistent personal attitude toward life or reality." He is, in other words, a person who can think or reason for himself and his philosophy will reflect the subjective truth of his own being. The person who is afraid to be different will subvert his reasoning to justify his conformity. The person who is afraid to be free will find reasons for his captivity. Instead of reason serving to relate man to the universe it becomes a weapon to deny him pleasure and enslave him to his misery.

It is in the name of reason that we distrust our instincts. Most people are convinced that if instinct were allowed to regulate behavior, the result would be disastrous. It is assumed that without the restraint of reason, the individual would run "wild." Does this mean that he would behave like a wild animal? Animals in the wild are not overeaters nor are they self-destructive in the way human beings are. They don't kill for political reasons and they don't suffer from the neuroses and psychoses that afflict civilized man.

Leslie Stephen in his *Science of Ethics* makes the statement that "instinct is reason limited to the immediate and incapable of reflecting on its own operations; and reason is an extended instinct, apprehending the distant and becoming conscious of its own modes of action" (p. 60). This view of the relationship between instinct and reason refutes the idea of a conflict between them. Reason, according to Stephen, furthers the aims of the instinctual drives (in line with Freud's concept of the reality principle). This principle states that an immediate gratification may be postponed or a present pain tolerated for the sake of a greater pleasure or to avoid a greater pain in the future. The reality principle extends the pleasure principle to the future.

Yet conflict arises because anxiety about the future overwhelms considerations of pleasure. Security rather than pleasure is the conscious objective of most people and security demands a constant vigilance. The postponement of pleasure takes on an indefinite character without one's realizing it. Since there is no absolute security, people live in a constant state of fear, a situation that would drive one "wild," i.e., mad if it were not supported by "reasons."

Parents reason with children mostly to stop them from following their natural impulses. The assumption is that because the parents have a reason they must be right. When a mother says to a child, "Don't run, you may fall and get hurt," she feels justified. Unfortunately, a young child lacks the ability to say, "I may not fall and you stop me because you are anxious." The use of reasons creates a state of right and wrong and since parents are superior reasoners, it always puts the child in the wrong.

The use of reasons (falsely called reasoning) forces a child to turn against his feelings. Suppose Johnny balks at stopping his play to accompany his mother on a visit to Aunt Ellen. He may say,

"I don't want to go. I don't like Aunt Ellen."

"But Aunt Ellen is a nice person," his mother replies. The conversation may continue as follows:

"I don't like Aunt Ellen."

"Aunt Ellen is your aunt."

"I don't like Aunt Ellen."

"But Aunt Ellen gave you a toy for Christmas."

"I don't like Aunt Ellen."

"You're a naughty boy and you're coming any way."

It would be much better to say to the child, "I can't leave you alone so you have to come."

Everybody has his reasons for acting as he does. To each person his reasons seem right because they derive from his feelings. A reason that is not based on a feeling is non-sense, that is, not sensing. The true reasons for our actions are our feelings. If we cut off our feelings, that is, if we deny our feelings to ourselves, they become projected onto others. If, for example, I am envious and do not sense my own envy, I will think that other people are envious of me. The way this works out is: I am in discomfort (pain) because I cannot accept my own feeling of envy. I do not understand my pain because I do not sense my envy. To account for my discomfort, I assume that it is due to envy but I believe that other people are envious of me. The thinking is right—the discomfort is due to envy; the sensing is wrong—I am out of touch with my feelings. Such reasoning, based as it is on a false premise, cannot be corrected by the rules of logic.

Reasons are like the paint on a canvas and it isn't the paint but the picture that counts. The picture provides certain sense impressions. It can be described as beautiful or ugly. It will strike one as beautiful if it is pleasurable, that is, exciting and also holds out a vision of happiness. If it does this, a person will feel it to be true, that is, in harmony and accord with the subjective truth of his body. What other criterion of truth does an individual have within himself than that it makes him feel good?

One cannot justify feelings by reasons since feelings, themselves, are the true reasons. In the final analysis, pleasure is the reason for living.

The Voice of the Body

6

Sex and Personality:
A Study in Orgastic Potency

LECTURE I: SEX AND PERSONALITY

If we had been interested in filling this auditorium, we would have entitled this series "How to Achieve Sexual Fulfillment in Four Easy Lectures." I would have had little hesitation in doing so if I could advise you how to achieve that goal. Unfortunately, sexual fulfillment cannot be realized through study or practice or the use of any special physical technique. Rather, it is the expression of a way of life, the sexual response of a mature personality. So if I must disappoint any expectations you may have had in this direction, I may be able to satisfy your need for an understanding of sexuality which will help you to avoid the confusion which envelops this subject in our culture.

No attempt can be made in these brief lectures to prove the concepts and statements offered. They are presented to set forth a broader view of sexuality than is found in the current literature on sex. They aim to create an attitude which regards sexuality as an expression of the spirit as much as an expression of the body.

These lectures are intended also to combat a tendency current among sexologists to treat sexual behavior as a kind of performance, the skills of which can be learned from books or developed through practice. Is sex a game in which the object is to "have fun"? Is the vaginal orgasm a myth? Is simultaneous climax an illusion? Is sexual fulfillment and happiness a dream? Have we reached the point where "anything goes" but nothing comes off? If there is one thing we can be sure of, it is that the degree of sexual unhappiness among people today is in direct proportion to the degree of so-called sexual sophistication.

The material presented in these lectures embodies the knowledge I have acquired in fifteen years of active psychiatric work and twenty years of study of this subject. It derives from the very common observation that a person's emotional problems and his sexual problems reflect the same disturbance in his personality. To think otherwise would imply that there are two compartments in a person's life: one compartment for his daytime functions (in the light, with his clothes on), and another for his functions in bed (in the dark, with the clothes off). My experience is that people are not so split. It shall be our contention that the sexual behavior of a person reflects his personality just as his personality is an expression of his sexual feelings.

Despite a common attempt to create the impression that one can function differently on these two levels, the fact is that the compulsive housewife is not a gay little nighttime moth, nor is the responsible executive a dashing lothario. When it comes to the sexual response, this compulsive housewife is afraid to let go, and the responsible executive is afraid to get involved.

The way you function sexually is the way you are. The kind of orgasm you can have sexually depends upon the kind of person you are. This is the theme that runs through the four lectures.

With this introduction we can proceed to the first lecture, which aims to establish the theoretical basis for this viewpoint.

The first important question that comes up is the relation of sex to love. Recently I wrote an article for the *Encyclopedia of Sexual Behavior* entitled "Movement and Feeling in Sex." There I stated that "there is no sex possible without love." I sent a copy of this article to the editor of a Catholic journal who had expressed an interest in my work. He wrote that he was impressed with the ideas in the article but that he could not quite accept the view that sex was an expression of love. He asked how I could reconcile this with the behavior of men who visit prostitutes or soldiers who rape women.

Now, I did not say that sex and love were the same thing. Love is regarded as a feeling, sex as an action. It is one of the contradictions in our cultured way of living that very frequently an action and the feeling it is intended to express are quite dissimilar. How many mothers have beaten their children in the name of love? How many husbands have been henpecked by loving wives? And yet it would be hard to affirm that the mother had no love for her children, nor the wife for her husband.

Psychological theory teaches us that sex, like other actions, often becomes a vehicle for expression of secondary drives which distort its primary function. To understand the relationship of sex to love, let us look at some of the biological phenomena which underlie the sexual response. Theoretically, a man cannot engage in the sexual act without an erection. And he cannot have an erection unless his genital organ becomes tumescent with blood. This blood comes from the heart, which has been described in popular language as the fountainhead of love. Just as tumescence is necessary for the male sexual function, congestion is necessary for the woman's sexual response. The sense of fullness in vagina and clitoris, the flow of the lubricating secretion, the feeling of heat, depend on the flow of blood from the heart to the pelvic area of the female. A woman's sexual receptivity is as much an expression of love as the physical desire of the man manifested by the erect phallus. If this were not so, no honest or decent person would speak of coitus as an act of love.

From another point of view, the psychological one, we can arrive at the same conclusion. Love may be defined as a feeling which impels the loving person to closeness with the loved object. This is true of the love between parents and children, friends, brothers, a man and a woman, and love between a man and the symbols and physical objects he cherishes. Love impels toward closeness, both in spirit (identification) and physically (contact and union). We want to be close to the people we love.

In what way is sex different? Sex brings people even closer together. If one does not separate the physical from the spiritual (and they can only be separated artificially when one discusses human behavior), sex brings people together spiritually as well as physically. Of course, the togetherness in sex is between man and woman, but this must be recognized as a basic form of togetherness.

If it is true that sex is an expression of love, we will have to revise our ideas about the sexual function. For one thing, the pleasure experienced in the sexual act must have some relation to the feeling of love between the two sexual partners. And the problem of unsatisfactory sexual relationships must be related either to the lack of feelings of love or to the inability to express those feelings in appropriate action.

It is difficult to conceive how the practice of special sexual techniques or manipulation procedures can significantly affect an individual's sexual response or pleasure. The opposite view, that sex is a performance which requires special skills, is set forth by Ellis in the following words:

> The technique of caressing your mate's clitoris or penis should be given special attention. Usually it is important to maintain steady and fairly prolonged clitoral contact, since many women complain that their husbands keep losing contact with their clitorises and that they are therefore continually frustrated and brought back to scratch after they had once begun and become aroused. In some instances, however, the clitoris may be intimately plucked, somewhat in the manner that a banjo string is plucked, or firmly pushed from side to side, again and again, until the female reaches new heights of excitement (and perhaps achieves a new orgasm with each new plucking.) Albert E. Ellis, *The Art and Science of Love.*

What about the evident exceptions to the statement that sex is an expression of love? Do I mean to say that a man loves the prostitute with whom he has relations? Yes. Many men have even married prostitutes.

Not infrequently a man feels free to express his love only to women whom he regards as inferior.

Then how explain the rapist? Is not his sexuality an expression of sadism rather than love? To analyze pathological sexual behavior would require volumes. I shall have to limit my comments on this problem to the observation that sadistic behavior is only directed toward those we love. It manifests the pathological condition of ambivalence: love and hate directed toward the same object. To the extent that the expression of love is inhibited, distorted or encumbered with secondary drives, the sexual response or function is limited in its pleasure and satisfaction.

If you accept the idea that sex is an expression of love, would you be willing to go along with the idea that love is an expression of sex? That love derives from sex? To support this concept, we would have to extend the range of our thinking and introduce ideas that may seem to lack scientific support.

Love, as we know it, is a relative newcomer in the field of emotions. By contrast, sex appeared early in the evolutionary scheme. There was sexual differentiation and sexual activity before there was anything among the animals which we could recognize as affection and love. Even the basic feelings of mother-love toward offspring are completely absent among most species of fish. Yet sex, as it functions among fish in mating and reproduction, is not so vastly different from sexual functions among higher animals, including man.

As one follows the sexual evolution of the animals, it is interesting to note that as the physical closeness or physical intimacy increases between the sexes, signs of tenderness and affection appear. In the mating of fish, the male hovers over the spot where the female has laid her eggs to discharge his sperms. In this process there is little physical contact between male and female. Contact during sexual activity is evident among the amphibian. The male frog, for example, will clasp the female with the pads of his forelegs as he covers her during discharge of the sexual gametes. Both eggs and sperms are discharged freely into the water where fertilization takes place.

There is neither penetration nor deposit of sperm cells into the body of the female until the evolution of the animals that live entirely on dry land. Perhaps there was no need of sexual penetration among the water-animals. The sea was the great repository, the great mother-substance. Ferenczi expressed the idea that sexual penetration for the land-animals has the function of providing a fluid medium of approximately the same chemical composition as the sea for the processes of fertilization and embryonic development. Whatever the reason, the fact is that the evolutionary development of the animals is characterized by a closer, more intimate and deeper sexual contact.

With the increase in physical closeness and physical intimacy which characterizes the sexual act among the mammals, there is the appearance of behavior which reflects feelings of affection, tenderness and love. Actions which have an affectionate quality can be observed among mammals that are sexually attracted to each other. When one observes this behavior, one is impressed by the close relation of affection to sexual feeling. But one may also see the opposite. Biting, scratching and similar actions are part of the sexual behavior of some mammals. This is most evident where the sexual pattern is one of male dominance and female submissiveness.

The human animal is no different. Among human beings, tenderness and affection between the sexes are commonly associated with sexual interest or they may lead to sexual desire.

Evolutionary development is characterized not only by an increase in the physical closeness and intimacy between the sexes, but also between mother and infant. Among those animals who deposit their eggs in the water or in the ground to hatch unattended, there are no signs of maternal love. Among the higher animals where the biological processes call for a closer physical relationship between mother and offspring, evidence of maternal love or tenderness appears. In the case of the mammalian female, who nourishes her young directly with her own body, we have the clearest evidence of maternal affection. But even maternal love, which is frequently taken as the example of pure love, has its origin in earlier physical intimacy of a sexual nature of which the child is the result.

Can love be defined as the consciousness of the desire for closeness and intimacy? Such a definition would include all forms of love: the dependent love of an infant for its mother and the sexual love of a man for a woman. It would have the advantage of relating the emergence of this emotion to the evolution and development of consciousness in general. Can we not say simply: that as consciousness evolved and the animal became aware of his need and desire for closeness with another organism, he experienced (perceptually) the feeling of longing which is at the basis of love. With the further development of consciousness to the point where the individual could anticipate the fulfillment of his longing, he developed the capacity to feel and to know love.

Love derives from the consciousness of the other as an object with whom physical contact and intimacy would lead to pleasure and satisfaction. Just as much as a child enjoys being held, so much does the mother enjoy holding the child. But since the feeling of love depends on the consciousness of the relationship, it will be increased by whatever increases our awareness of the other person. The change in the coital position from the rear approach employed by most mammals to the frontal approach used by most men increased our awareness of the other person. It is conceivable that this change heightened our consciousness of love. (It is interesting in this connection to note that whereas most primitive mothers carry their infants on their backs, the civilized mother, who is perhaps more conscious of her relationship to her child, tends to hold it in the face-to-face position.)

It may surprise one to learn that some people deny the obvious and immediate relationship of sex to love, and love to sex. If love is consciously experienced in the sexual relationship, the sexual excitation is increased and the sexual pleasure in climax is greater. This is to be expected since the greater the desire, the greater the pleasure in its fulfillment. But love also arises from sex; that is, as a result of sexual pleasure, one not infrequently develops strong love feelings for another person. I have no hesitating in stating that sexual activity without any conscious feeling of attraction to the other person produces little pleasure and is relatively unsatisfying.

Representation of coitus in the two positions

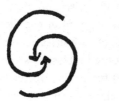 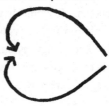

a) Rear approach, male covering female b) Front approach, face to face
Fig. 1

The relationship between sex and love may be set forth as follows: Sex, divorced from its conscious correlates, that is, as an instinctual drive, obeys the pleasure-principle. The build-up of sexual tension would lead to an immediate attempt to discharge it with the nearest available object. But where love enters the scene, the reality-principle becomes operative. Knowing love, one is aware that the pleasure of the sexual discharge can be heightened by certain objects or lowered by others. One learns to hold back the action, to consciously restrain the discharge of the sexual tension, until the most favorable situation is available, namely, a loved object. This awareness of selectivity in the choice of a sexual object in the interest of a greater sexual pleasure is one of the main functions of love. And since one looks for a special object, one becomes more conscious of the object, more aware of the other, more sensitive to the love partner.

These few remarks can do no more than sketch the relationship of love to sex. We must leave many questions unanswered. How can we explain, for example, the case where the love feelings (tenderness, affection, etc.) are directed toward one person while the sexual desire is directed toward another? Or the situation in which sexual desire diminishes as one experiences greater love and tenderness for the sexual object? These conditions are the result of neurotic disturbances of the personality which, unfortunately, are beyond the scope of these lectures except insofar as they can be discussed incidentally to our main theme.

To attempt to define the relationship of sex to personality, we must go further back along the great chain of life than the fish, to life in the form of the single celled animal or plant. Among the one-cell organisms, life can be reproduced in two ways: asexually or sexually. In the asexual mode, reproduction is by cell division or by a process known as budding. An amoeba, for example, will divide into two daughter cells when it reaches a certain size or state of maturity. The resulting two amoebas then proceed to grow and mature. When they in turn reach full size, they divide into four daughter cells. This process can apparently go on indefinitely so long as the conditions for life and growth of the amoeba are favorable.

An amoeba need never die. By means of cell division it rejuvenates by becoming two younger amoebas. Since seemingly nothing is added or lost in the process of cell division, the old amoeba is identical with the two daughter cells. So in a sense the amoeba is immortal. But by the same token, since the two daughter cells are identical, their offspring will be identical and the amoeba will have no individuality. It is unimportant whether one amoeba is absolutely identical with another or not. The statement that the asexual mode of reproduction, whether by cell division or by budding, makes no allowance or provision for the phenomenon of individuality is valid.

Among the protozoa there is an organism which is more highly differentiated in its body structure than the amoeba. It is called Volvox and it is known as the "roller" because of its spinning movement as it travels through the fluid medium. Volvox has developed a sexual mode of reproduction in addition to the asexual form. After several generations in which reproduction takes place by asexual means, a sexual generation arises. Some of the little organisms will produce egg cells which are extruded from the body. Others produce male gametes or sperm cells which are also extruded from the body. When male and female gametes meet, they fuse to become the origin of another Volvox.

But the parent cell which has extruded the male or female gametes from its body has by this process completed its life. It dies. It drops quietly to the bottom, stops all movement, and dies. As one zoologist expressed it, "This is the first advent of natural death in the animal kingdom, and all for the sake of sex."

The amoeba never just dies. It can die if there is no food or water, or if the temperature of the water is too high or too low. You cannot easily crush it; it is too small. But there is no natural death among the amoeba. Volvox dies naturally; it comes to the end of a span of existence and ceases to be. And in the sense that it has an existence, limited in time, and therefore unique, it is an individual.

The uniqueness of Volvox has another basis which the sexual mode of reproduction provides. When male and female gametes fuse, the fertilized egg is endowed with hereditary traits contributed by the sperm as well as those originally its own. Half of its chromosomes come from one parent, half from another. The process is such that the resulting organism is different from any other organism that exists or has existed. Sexual reproduction facilitates a thorough reshuffling of hereditary patterns and produces organisms which are unique in space and time, as we can observe among the higher animals.

It would be a mistake to assume that death is the price the organism pays for sex. It is true that death enters the stage of life from one wing while sexuality enters from the other. But the process which introduces sex and natural death is the process of individuation.

Let us examine the evolutionary picture again. We have said that the amoeba is immortal, at least potentially. It is immortal because it has no unique structure to its protoplasm. It cannot develop a unique structure since this would not survive the process of cell-division. For the same reason, it cannot develop those structural differentiations which make the higher forms of life possible. Imagine dividing a man in half so that you would get two identical men! Or try it with a fish, a crab, or even a worm. If specialized structures were to develop at the same time that the individual life itself was to continue to go on, the reproductive function had to be divorced from the over-all functions of the organism. A mode of reproduction had to be developed in which small portions of the organism were set aside for this particular purpose while the total structure of the organism could remain intact over a period of time.

Sex is not the cause of death. Quite the opposite. Death is often related to the loss of sexual feeling or libido. Death comes at the end of a sexual life, not because of one. One old Indian of 104 years stated this succinctly when asked the explanation of his long life. His advice was: "Plenty of hard physical work—but retain your interest in the opposite sex."

Speaking metaphysically, one can say that death is the result of the inability of the organism to sustain and move the increasing structure which life creates. Age is characterized by the loss of flexibility and elasticity. While this is true, its converse is more meaningful. The experience of life is structured into the organism, reducing its motility and available energy. Advancing age is increasing rigidity as death is rigor mortis. To appreciate this, one has only to compare the body of a young person with the body of an older one.

These relationships can be shown diagrammatically:

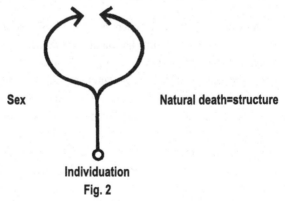

Sex   **Natural death=structure**

Individuation
Fig. 2

This may be clear so far, but we have ignored an important question. Why does the amoeba have to divide in the first place? What force moves life onward to bigger and more complex structural forms? What is the power of the drive to individuation? These questions pose for us the problem of the nature of life.

May I offer one idea which will clarify our understanding of the sexual function. For example, crystals in a solution grow by the addition of substance to the outside; the crystal becomes larger. But in life, growth occurs from the center outward. As the amoeba grows, he runs into a difficulty. His insides grow faster than his membrane. His protoplasmic mass increases in geometric proportion while his surface increases arithmetically. Soon he reaches the point where the inner pressure exerted outward threatens to become greater than the surface tension of the membrane. The amoeba must find some way to reduce the internal pressure, or he will burst. Cell division accomplishes this reduction of tension beautifully. It reduces the mass by two at the same time that it increases the surface area.

Life itself is characterized by the process of producing excess energy, that is, energy above the needs of the organism for survival. This production of excess energy is exemplified in the fact that a fish may produce one million eggs; a tree, one thousand apples; a cat, one hundred kittens in its lifetime, etc. The excess energy makes possible the growth of the organism.

But when growth has reached its natural limits, some other means of using the excess energy must be found. In the lower animals, this takes the form of the asexual modes of reproduction: cell division, budding, and the production of vegetative daughter cells. In the higher animals, where the individual structure has to be maintained, this excess energy is channeled into the discharge of sexual substances via the sexual function.

It is interesting to note in this connection that the sexual function does not take over until the organism has reached its full growth. Even more striking is the parallel between the convulsion of the sexual orgasm and the convulsion which an amoeba undergoes in cell division. If one has seen the latter in cinemicrophotography, one is impressed by the intensity of the reaction. Its ability to discharge tension cannot be doubted.

Seen in this light, the sexual drive is an expression of the life force in the organism. The more excess energy an organism produces, the stronger is the drive for sexual discharge. But this same excess energy is what creates growth and personality; that is, the same excess energy is available for growth, the development of personality, or sexuality, depending on the life cycle of the organism or its biological needs. We can, therefore, substitute new terms in Figure 2.

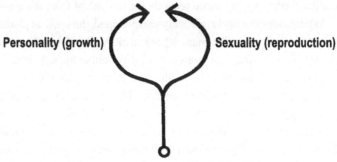

Personality (growth)   **Sexuality (reproduction)**

Life process—process of individuation

Fig. 3

The relationships portrayed in this diagram are to be interpreted as follows: the process of individuation is the life process itself by virtue of its production of excess energy. This excess energy is channeled into the antithetical functions of personality and sex. The function of sexuality includes that of reproduction. Quantitatively these two functions are equal, since both derive from the same excess energy. This means that if the personality is vital and alive, the sexuality of the individual will show the same qualities. Conversely, if the personality is dead, the sexuality is equally dead. Qualitatively, too, sexuality reflects personality and also undermines it. A rigid person's sexual function is just as rigid as his personality. A person whose behavior is designed to impress another will have a sexual function which is designed to impress another.

In addition to the foregoing interpretation, Diagram 3 offers us some interesting ideas about the relation of sex and anxiety. We have postulated the concept that sex and personality are antithetical functions which arise through the process of individuation and as a result of the operation of the life forces. The functions which are associated with the development of personality create in the individual a sense of his uniqueness, a feeling of his "apartness", and the condition of "aloneness." This is supported by the experience of any individual whose personality is sufficiently developed; that is, the stronger the personality, the greater the individuality and the more separate the individual from the mass.

Where individuality is relatively undeveloped, the sense of aloneness does not occur. Primitive man, whose identity was determined by his membership in a tribe, was rarely conscious of either his individuality or his isolation. An amoeba is never alone. It exists as part of a continuous flow of life from one amoeba to another. The lower organisms all show this phenomenon of being part of the natural order—one with their environment. But the lower animals have no feeling of their individuality. The more individual we become, the more alone we sense ourselves, the more isolated we feel ourselves. Personality by definition creates uniqueness, difference, isolation.

Many psychologists are of the opinion that this isolation, this sense of being unique which is the concomitant of our individual personalities, is the underlying cause of the anxiety with which civilized man struggles. Certainly nothing creates more anxiety than the feeling of being alone, apart, isolated. This theory, advanced by Rollo May, has much to support it.

What is the antidote to this destructive anxiety? Our diagram suggests that while personality is a function which tends to separate people, sexuality is the biological function which tends to bring them together. We have previously described sexuality as a natural force which leads to closeness, to identification, to union with the "other."

According to the diagram, life creates two forces, one which tends to apartness and individuality, the other to merger and loss of individuality. It would be very easy to describe this second force as love, and it is love. But it is love in action; and love in action, as we saw earlier, is sex.

The fact is that no man who is in bed with a woman he loves or cares for ever feels alone. It does not matter what situation he happens to be in—he can be a stranger in a foreign land, an enemy in hostile territory—but when he is in bed with a woman, he never feels alone. And even without the woman, as long as the sex drive is imperative, as long as it is conscious and free of guilt, the anxiety of aloneness is not experienced.

If it is correct to relate anxiety to the condition of "isolation," being alone, it is equally correct to relate it to the failure of the sexual feelings in the individual to prevent anxiety. In this sense it can be seen as valid as the modern sociological view which relates anxiety to interpersonal difficulties.

Sexuality determines personality, since it determines the individual's relationship to the other and to the world. We saw earlier that love derived from the sexual feelings, that sexuality was the force which urged to closeness and intimacy with another. The sexual person is a loving person and a joyful person, as we shall see in Lecture III. His sexuality provides both the main source of his pleasure and satisfaction in life and a positive orientation toward others and toward the world. In the same way, the bitter person is invariably a sexually frustrated person. Similarly, the depressed person is suffering from the depression of his sexual drive, probably cause by repeated failures and disappointments.

We can go one step further. Personality is not limited to the psychic functions of the individual. Since it denotes the quality of the person, it refers to his physical quality as well as his psychic qualities. Therefore we can anticipate that the sexuality of a person is reflected in his body as well as his mind.

Nothing new about this, you may say. And you are right. What is new is the ability to understand the language of the body so that we can correctly interpret what we see. Without this knowledge one can easily be misled into confusing the symbol with the reality. Marilyn Monroe was a symbol of sexuality, not the embodiment of it. The reason is that her body lacked integration, unity. A body without unity reflects the lack of fusion of the pregenital drives and the absence of a strong unifying genital drive. "Jello on wheels," as Jack Lemmon called her in "Some Like It Hot."

What are the physical characteristics of the sexually mature personality? The answer has to be simple: a body that is harmonious, integrated, coordinated, and alive. In two words, a body that is beautiful and graceful in its normal and natural situation.

These ideas enable us to separate the chaff from the wheat in sexual matters. We cannot be duped by statements or pretenses of sexual prowess. The proof is in the pudding. The sexuality of a person is in his being. His sexual fulfillment is in his over-all good feeling, joyfulness, and happiness. In the next lecture we shall apply these concepts to the problem of homosexuality as opposed to heterosexuality.

Let us briefly summarize. We say that sexuality reflects personality and personality mirrors the sexuality of an individual. The relationship is an indirect one in that each is a product of the vitality of aliveness of the organism. The more alive the organism is, the more vibrant is its personality and the more intense is its sexual drive. Each is a direct expression of the energy or vitality of the organism.

Sex does not create personality since neither sexual sophistication nor sexual techniques increase the vitality, they cannot further the development of personality. But this is not to say that sexuality has no effect on personality. Since sexuality provides one of the main sources of pleasure and joy in life, any limitation or inhibition upon sexual feelings will depress the vital, energetic processes of the body and so adversely affect personality.

The emphasis is upon sexual *feeling*, not sexual "acting out." The latter, which includes sexual promiscuity, is the expression of a *lack* of sexual feeling. Such behavior denotes the frantic or hysterical search for sexual feeling and is doomed to disappointment by the very condition which created the need.

Psychologists recognize that personality is closely related to the individual's ability to love and to receive or accept love. Individuals in whom this capacity is highly developed have a positive attitude towards life, a feeling for closeness and identification with another being, and the ability to express this feeling in appropriate action which can bring about effectual discharge and thus gratify the instinct.

LECTURE II:
HOMOSEXUALITY AND HETEROSEXUALITY

In the first lecture we expressed the idea that, aside from some of the simplest single-celled organisms, life is basically sexual. And that by virtue of its sexuality, life develops the uniqueness which we call personality. Perhaps we should say that sex is an expression of life, but it would be equally true to say that life is a product of sex. If this statement seems broad, we need only remember that life arises through the sexual act of creation.

We set forth the thesis that sex reflects the personality of the individual and the personality mirrors the sexuality of the individual. In this lecture we shall study the application of this thesis to the problem of homosexuality. We also stated that sex is a manifestation of love, and that its meaning must be sought in the feelings which motivate sexual behavior.

This view challenges a current concept that sex is a performance and that a person's ability to love is equal to his ability to perform. The very term "perform" implies an action which is designed to impress others with the skill or technique of the performer. One performs to create an effect, not to express his feelings. When a patient complains that his sexual performance was a failure, he betrays his neurotic attitude to sexuality. If he loved his partner and was able to express that love in his sexual activity, this experience of the sexual contact would be highly pleasurable and satisfactory. In the absence of such a result, one must question one's feelings or one's ability to express them.

Another current concept at variance with the ideas we expressed earlier is that sex is "fun." To say that sex is fun is to regard sexual activity as play, as a game in which "anything goes." Perhaps this explains why the homosexual is called a "gay" person. In some respects he "plays" at sex like a pre-adolescent, as we shall see later. But the homosexual is gay; he is certainly neither happy nor joyful. Under analysis he proves to be one of the most tragic figures of our times.

But the phenomenon of homosexuality is much more complicated than this. We tend to think that sex represents the difference between male and female, or pertains to that difference, yet there are many sexual activities that seem to have no relation to that difference. For example, the physical act of masturbation does not seem to involve the concept of male and female, since it can be conceived as an activity which is limited to one's own body. Homosexuality seems to deny that the difference is important.

Homosexuality poses an enigma. It raises the question whether there are two sexes or three (including the homosexual), or whether man is basically bisexual so that he can be either heterosexual or homosexual.

One interesting thing is the intense reaction which homosexuality arouses in people, the so-called normal people. On the one hand, they frequently express considerable antagonism and hostility toward homosexuals. On the other hand, they manifest a certain fascination and interest in homosexual practices. One sees this in the influx of tourists to the "gay" bars in Greenwich Village. These people expose themselves to the homosexual atmosphere at the same time that they express their repugnance and anger against it. It seems that the horror some people have about homosexuality reflects their fear that they may be tainted with the "disease."

When one attempts to study homosexuality as a sociological phenomenon, one finds that it is almost universal. It can be found in the animal kingdom, in many different cultures, and to some extent, so far as we know, it has existed at all times in our own culture. One must wonder then: is it a natural thing? A different thing that can exist side by side with heterosexuality?

Another enigma is the fact (which one cannot deny) that the homosexual is frequently found in the forefront of cultural activity—in the theater, the arts, music, design, the dance, and so many other creative activities. Certainly this must have something to do with the social forces in a culture such as ours which places an exaggerated value on so-called aggression, so-called virility, competitiveness, drive, success.

The heterosexual is discouraged from those activities which depend upon emotional expression and therefore seem passive and feminine. The homosexual who eschews the competitive struggle is only too happy to have the creative field as his personal terrain. But surely this cannot be the whole answer. It must also be due to the fact that the competitive struggle is so severe, so fierce, that it leaves the normal individual who engages in it with little energy or inclination for the pursuit of artistic interests.

Society's role in homosexuality is complex. To explore its influence in this problem is beyond the scope of this lecture. It is significant to us that while male homosexuality is almost universally condemned, female homosexuality is tolerated. Thus there have been laws penalizing the male homosexual; there are no such laws punishing female homosexuality.

This attitude must have at its base the fear that homosexuality in a man represents a condition of weakness, a lack of strength, an impotence. Such a strong condemnation can proceed only from an inner feeling that the society or culture depends upon its aggressive structure to survive. In terms of the values of our culture, the homosexual is regarded as an inferior being. The question then arises as to whether he really is inferior. Is there any truth in this social assumption?

To gain some clarity in this discussion, we must make a fundamental distinction between a homosexual experience and the homosexual attitude. The experience which is engaged in for convenience, that is, in the absence of the opposite sex, is found in the animal kingdom, in all cultures, and at all times. Those who participate in such an activity do not deny their preference for the heterosexual relationship. All it tells us is that the sex drive can be so potent, so imperative, that it overrides the appearance of reality.

The homosexual attitude is the subject of this lecture. This is characterized by a preference for sexual experience with the same sex. Perhaps the homosexual attitude can be defined as one in which the individual's sexual drive is not oriented toward the opposite sex or, better, that it is oriented away from the opposite sex.

In the preceding lecture I remarked that the sexual drive could be viewed as the biological force which functions to overcome the sense of aloneness and of isolation which the process of individuation creates. Sexuality brings people together, not only the two sexual partners, but large numbers, in such activities as parties, festivals, dances, celebrations, all of which are oriented to the pleasure of sexuality. Sexuality is so closely related to the problem of loneliness that sexual frustration and the feeling of being alone are experienced as similar qualities. Conversely, sexual fulfillment and the feeling of belonging are also experienced as closely related qualities. Later we shall examine this relationship more fully.

At this point I should like to introduce a concept which has an important bearing on this subject. Individuality is not only associated with the feeling of aloneness, it is also accompanied by a sense of incompleteness. The sexual urge to union is not only an urge for self-completion. It is as if the self is fully realized only in sexual union through which the isolation of individuality is overcome.

This concept is similar to a myth credited to Plato: man and woman were originally one being, one creature, which God split asunder to create the sexes. Ever since the two halves have been struggling to come together again to become the whole being. This myth may be interpreted also as an awareness that life once functioned on an asexual level.

The feeling of incompleteness as related to sexuality is dramatically illustrated in certain dreams, fantasies or actions. I refer to the desire or the attempt by a man to take his own penis into his mouth and thereby satisfy and fulfill himself. This desire to be self-sufficient, complete unto one's self, independent of the need for a woman, is found in neurotic males who have some unconscious fear of the female. But the fantasy or action in which this desire expresses itself represents an early primitive state in the history of the individual when such self-sufficiency seemed to exist. Actually this early "primitive" state could be interpreted as representing two different periods: one in the history of the species, the other in the history of the specific individual.

The first period would correspond to a time in man's early development when the consciousness of self had not yet appeared. In this period of his evolution, man felt himself to be part of the universe, as the animal does, and neither incomplete nor isolated nor alone. The significant thing for us about this early period is that it is represented in stone tablets or other artifacts uncovered by archaeological investigations as a serpent with a tail in its mouth. Neumann describes this symbol as "the circular snake, the primal dragon of the beginning that bites its own tail, the self-begetting uroboros." As the Heavenly Serpent, the uroboros "slays, weds, and impregnates itself. It is man and woman, begetting and conceiving and giving birth, active and passive, above and below, at once."

The theory behind this symbol is that the serpent can eat his own tail and so generate himself out of his own substance, thereby being endless, infinite, and complete in itself. One wonders if the fantasy of taking one's own penis into one's own mouth does not recall this early state of consciousness.

The second period corresponds to the time in man's individual development when he existed in the "round" of which the circle is a symbol. In this state, the organism felt complete and self-contained, unconscious of need or effort. The symbol of the uroboros also represents the organism's early life in the womb as much as it represents man's earliest state of unconsciousness. Neumann writes: "The uroboros appears as the round 'container,' i.e., the maternal womb, but also as the union of masculine and feminine opposites. In the womb, the organism is curled up into itself, unaware of any lack in itself."

It is obvious that once the person is born, once he is out in the world, it is impossible to get back either to the womb or to a primal state of consciousness in which one is unaware of one's needs or one's isolation. There is no alternative but union with another individual and in this need the homosexual is no different from anyone else. He too needs union with another, both to complete his feeling of self and to gain a sense of belonging, of being part of the whole; in other words, he needs the feeling of loving and of being loved. His pattern differs from the normal in that his love-object is a person of the same sex. How should we interpret this anomaly?

Infantile sexuality as opposed to adult sexuality is characterized by a search for uroboric completion, that is, for fulfillment through self-love. This takes the form of masturbation in which the circle is completed via the contact of the hands with the genitals. The love-object of the homosexual is, on one level of consciousness, an image of himself. On this level, homosexuality has many of the attributes of masturbation, especially the concept of self-love. On another level, however, the homosexual is joining with another person in an attempt at a mature relationship.

I think that homosexuality can be viewed as a stage between the self-love of infancy and the adult love of heterosexuality. This type of sexual relationship is frequently found among pre-adolescents and early adolescents. Whether this relationship of young boys with each other involves sexual activity or not, it is a common step in the process of development of adult heterosexual love patterns. Homosexuality at this stage seems to be an arrested development.

In terms of the other, homosexuality is also an unconscious attempt to establish a heterosexual relationship. Theodor Reik made the observation, which I believe is true, that in a homosexual relation one of the partners unconsciously imagines that the other is of the opposite sex, even though he is conscious of the fact that he is not. In the homosexual activity, one of the partners takes the role of the opposite sex. Analysis of the homosexual relationship reveals that the homosexual partner is treated as if he were a symbol and representative of the woman and the mother. Even the act of masturbation reflects, on either a conscious or unconscious level, an awareness of the other sex. For the man, the hand represents the vagina; for the woman it represents the penis.

If the homosexual, in symbolic form, acts out the sexual relation in symbolic form, why is he unable to do so in reality? What stands in the way of or prevents a mature heterosexual activity by the homosexual? For the answers to these questions we have to turn to information gathered from the clinical and analytic investigations of homosexual feelings and behavior. One of the things that analytic investigation reveals is that the homosexual is afraid of the opposite sex. Related to this fear but on a deeper level are feelings of hostility toward the opposite sex. Since the fear is uppermost, it blocks off any possibility of expressing love-feelings directly towards the opposite sex. This would not be true if the feelings of hostility and anger were uppermost. In the latter case, sufficient aggression would be available to permit the carrying out of the heterosexual act.

The presence of fear and hostility on an unconscious level forces the child into an unconscious identification with the opposite sex. Unconscious identification, as W. Reich pointed out in *Character Analysis*, is always with the parent who was regarded as the most threatening figure. If we are to understand homosexuality we must know what kind of family situation or parental relationship constituted the soil in which the homosexual's personality developed.

The observations which I shall offer are not submitted as definitive statements of this problem. They are based upon my own clinical experience and upon the research of other analytic investigations. They are presented as a basis for our further discussion and not as positive proof of etiologic factors. With these qualifications in mind, I would state that male homosexuality has its origin in an incestuous relationship with the mother. I shall elaborate the pathological situation to show what I believe are the forces which impede the normal psychosexual development of the future homosexual.

It stands to reason, and clinical experience confirms the observation, that a mother who will develop an incestuous relationship with a child is an emotionally disturbed and immature individual. The basis for the incestuous attachment to the child is a lack of satisfaction and fulfillment in her sexual relations with her husband. The mature parent would cope with this problem directly. The emotionally disturbed and immature mother transfers her sexual longing to her son. This is not done consciously but is acted out in a variety of ways. The boy is frequently kept in his mother's company, exposed to her feelings, seduced into some seemingly innocuous physical intimacy, like helping her dress or undress, and discouraged from contact with other boys and girls. The mother of the homosexual has been described as C.B.I. – close-binding-intimate. She ties the child to her. Consciously the importance of the boy to his mother is reflected in her feeling that "This boy of mind will fulfill me." This is interpreted by the mother as her wish that the boy will be a great man, a hero, outstanding, and that people will point to his mother as the responsible agent. Unconsciously, however, this feeling has a sexual significance.

Invariably in these cases the boy takes the father's place in the mother's affections. Not infrequently, he is seduced into sharing the same bed with her. I have found that the result of this behavior is to create a sexual excitement in the boy, directed toward the mother, with which he cannot cope. On the one hand he cannot reject his mother; on the other, he cannot express his sexual feelings toward her. In fact, he is left with no choice but to cut off these feelings at the expense of deadening his body.

We can anticipate that the father in these family situations will be as neurotically disturbed as the mother. This is constantly being proved in analytic investigations of the family background of emotionally ill persons. The father's reactions to the mother's attitude will be one of hostility toward the boy. He will regard him as a competitor who threatens his own position. It is difficult to see how he can avoid this feeling, since the mother has forced the child into this role.

The father will also be negative—critical of the boy in self-defense, calling him a "sissy". And in truth the mother is making a sissy of the boy by alienating him from his father. But the odds are that the father will also be inadequate as a male figure with whom the boy can consciously identify and upon whom he can pattern his attitudes. The father's hostility makes it even more difficult for the boy to reject his mother. She becomes his protection against the hostile father.

The opposite attitude on the part of the mother can also force a child into a homosexual pattern of sexual responsivity. If she feels inferior and humiliated by her sexual role as a woman, she can project her feminine sexuality upon her son, reversing and acting out what she feels is the masculine contempt for woman. These are the phallic mothers who pride themselves upon their possession of the so-called masculine qualities of strength, aggression, and power.

These attitudes are, of course, unconscious. They are acted out by dressing the boy in little girl's clothes, babying him, being over-protective, discouraging self-assertion, etc. The mother takes the masculine role of being the strong one, the knowing one. The sexual implication of this reversal of roles is seen in certain anal practices. These mothers frequently give the child enemas, insert suppositories or other medication which have the symbolic significance of sexual intercourse in which the child plays the role of passive female. Not infrequently one finds both roles being acted out by the mother. At times she is phallic and aggressive; at others, seductive and dependent.

The strong feelings which parents have about the sex of the child are often expressed as early as the time of birth. The first thing which parents want to know about the newborn child is its sex. In their emotional reaction to the announcement that it is a boy or a girl, one can determine much about their future feelings toward the child.

We discussed the distortions which can exist in a mother's relation to a boy child. The same distortions can characterize her relations to a girl child. She can regard the newcomer as a future rival and competitor (unconsciously, of course) and in consequence make every effort to masculinize the little girl. This is done by reserving for herself the role of being the helpless, dependent and passive figure in the home. The little girl is forced to take on the responsibility for her mother's welfare which places her in the same position as her father. This is the theme of the wicked stepmother who is determined that the girl child will not dethrone her from her queenly position.

If the identification is with the father in this case, it is because he has betrayed the child in not affirming her femininity nor supporting her rights as a person against the mother. The fear of and hostility toward the father stem from the child's inability to express any warm, tender and pre-genital sexual feelings toward him. In part, too, the fear of and hostility toward the father result from transference of feelings from the mother to the father which is normal in every girl's development.

A disturbed mother can also project her own rejected female sexuality upon a girl child. This would have the effect of saying "You are the rejected inferior being. I am the superior one." A situation such as this is, as I have shown elsewhere, is often found to be of significant etiologic importance in the development of schizophrenia or the schizoid personality.

A woman who is unfulfilled sexually has to do something with her sexual feeling. It cannot be thrown away since it is part of her body. It cannot be talked away or denied. If it is not accepted, it will be projected generally onto the child. In fact I would not hesitate to say that children tend to act out their parents' unconscious sexual feelings and desires. This is tragic because no one knows what his unconscious holds. One is therefore powerless to guard against the phenomenon. Perhaps the only guaranty for healthy children is a satisfactory and fulfilling relationship between the parents.

Just as homosexuality results form the unconscious "acting out" by parents upon children, so homosexual activity is marked by the "acting out" by homosexuals upon each other of repressed feelings which the homosexual has toward his parents. No homosexual relationship is free from this tendency. Thus, the homosexual relationship is characterized by the ambivalence of love and hate, fear and hostility, dependency and resentment, submission and dominance. One can discern sadistic feelings by one partner against the other who is masochistically submissive. The masochistic submission has as one of its objectives the need to place the other party in the wrong in order to obtain some release of sexual feeling, while for the first party the sadistic behavior is necessary for some degree of sexual satisfaction.

Now let us look at the personality of the homosexual. There is enough clinical evidence to indicate on the psychological level that the homosexual feels himself to be a partially castrated individual. This is manifested by his preoccupation with genital feeling, betraying his fear and anxiety over the loss of genital sensation. The anxiety is shown in the constant awareness of the genitals and in a manner of dress and behavior which calls attention to them.

In bioenergetic analysis one finds that the homosexual is usually emotionally deadened. He may not lack creative intelligence or creative ideas, but there is a severe limitation in the range of emotional expressivity. Neither anger nor sadness is easily expressed, and such feelings as enthusiasm, disappointment and joy are often lacking.

The emotional deadness is paralleled by an unaliveness of the body. Skin tone and color are poor. Spontaneity in gesture and movement are absent. The motility of the body is markedly decreased. The bioenergetic charge of the organism, that is, its vitality, is noticeably reduced.

In view of these findings, we must revise our ideas about homosexual activity. It is less an expression of strong sexual drive based on sexual feeling than a need for sexual feeling and excitement. How does the homosexual get the excitement and feeling which he lacks? Strangely enough, he gets them by the same mechanism which was originally responsible for his problem, that is, by identification. In a homosexual encounter much of the excitement is derived from the reaction of the other partner. For this reason, the homosexual feels alive only in the homosexual experience.

The homosexual is like a lost, frightened child who is not crying simply because he is too shocked by the feeling of abandonment to cry. He clings to the homosexual partner as a lost child clings to its mother. At the same time, he wants some emotional reaction from the partner-mother to show that the latter feels his need and will respond to it. These feelings are transposed to the sexual level where they are acted out in combination with genital longing and desire. His behavior is determined by a strange mixture of uroboric elements and adult sexual feeling; that is, his action attempts to combine the desire for fulfillment and completion within oneself and the need for union with another person. It is said that in a homosexual relationship, two halves make one person.

One cannot approach the opposite sex with an inadequate sexual concept or sexual charge. To do so would only lead to failure and a further increase in the feeling of castration. And since the woman was the original seducer and castrator of the homosexual male, it is unlikely that he will risk what little feeling and contact he has with his genitals in a sexual relation with another woman whom he fears may do the same thing to him.

Actually there is a loss of penile feeling in satisfactory heterosexual experience. The genital organ goes through a cycle from fullness, erection and feeling to emptiness, flaccidity and no feeling. For the homosexual who is preoccupied with his genitals, this loss of genital feeling is equivalent to the loss of life. His genital feeling is his lifeline, and he cannot afford to reduce the genitals to impotence.

In a normal person, however, the loss of genital feeling is compensated by an increased feeling in the rest of the body. The orgastic discharge is characterized by the return flow of feeling into the body so that while the genitals lose sensation, the body gains increased aliveness and good feeling. Thus, at the same time the sexual charge is reduced, the sexual image of the body is enhanced. As a result the sexual identity and the personality of the individual are strengthened. In the homosexual experience, the genitals do not lose feeling. On the contrary, the homosexual contact leaves the genital organs with more feeling than before; the homosexual is more conscious of his genital organ and therefore less anxious about it.

In the normally healthy male, sexuality has a double aspect. The primary sexual feeling is related to the body, and only secondarily is the genital organ involved. This dual aspect is expressed in our way of speaking. The French, for example, describe the penis as "mon petit frere," my little brother. We frequently call it by name, Peter or Johnny. The normal male has himself and his "little brother." The homosexual has only a "Peter" and hangs onto him for dear life.

In a recent study of homosexuality by a group of psychoanalytic doctors, the authors made several statements about the physical appearance and motility of the homosexual which are pertinent to our discussion. I quote:

> When these gesture-voice affectations are taken on by effeminate males the motoric pattern does not suggest freedom of movement but gives the appearance of constriction and inhibition, since the movements are confined to small arcs in space; they are directed inwardly towards the midline of the body rather than away from it...The effeminate behavior noted among some homosexuals appears to us as neither 'masculine' nor 'feminine'-it is sui generis, i.e., it expresses some caricaturing of female mannerisms but is set within a behavioral framework of motoric constriction and inhibition.

In another context the authors comment about a group of adolescent homosexuals studied at Bellevue Hospital:

> The effeminate adolescents related comfortably to other effeminate homosexuals and to lesbians and women considered as asexual, but became very anxious in the presence of a female perceived as 'sexual'...One such patient spent the night in the home of his girl friend when her parents were away. She came to his bed dressed only in pajamas and lay down next to him. He became 'numb,' 'without feeling,' 'paralyzed.' Within a few days he yielded to a compulsive urge to go to Greenwich Village bar and pick up a homosexual.

We know that the body of the homosexual individual cannot tolerate strong heterosexual feelings. It fights them by "going dead," i.e., becoming numb and without feeling. The homosexual act is a reaction to this loss of feeling; it is an attempt to regain genital sensation.

How does heterosexuality compare with homosexuality? It would be simple to say that homosexuality is the union of the like or similar—heterosexuality is the union of the different or opposites. However, we have learned that behind every homosexual act is the unconscious image of sexual union with the opposite sex. Could we expect that under the façade of heterosexuality, one or both of the partners may act out homosexual attitudes and feelings? Let us explore this idea.

We saw that the homosexual feeling derives much of its charge from identification. It is in part a vicarious experience. This also happens in many heterosexual relationships. The man whose excitement is dependent on the woman's excitement, whose pleasure derives from her satisfaction, is acting out a homosexual attitude. This kind of sexual behavior reflects identification with the woman which denies the man's different and opposite nature. This attitude characterizes the man who knows more about female sexuality than he does about his own, who is less interested in his own feelings than in the woman's. One can easily rationalize such an attitude as empathy and understanding; however, it denies the antithetical nature of the sexes.

Another homosexual concept which can be found in heterosexual activities is the concept of service. The homosexual "services" his partner and it is frequently so described. But this is what a man does whose primary concern is heterosexual activity is to bring the woman to climax. Similarly the compulsion to have sexual relations with a woman simply because she is excited betrays the need to "service" the woman. Under the banner of the art of love, many sexologists advocate a sex technique which is based upon the concept of "service" to each other. Ellis, for example, writes: "The deeply empathic individual not only passively notes what his or her bed mate requires but actively *looks for, seeks out* this mate's requirements and then caters to them." (author's italics). I have always believed that the sexual relation was the union of equals, each of whom was competent to take care of his or her own needs. The above quotation makes each partner the servant of the other.

It appears to be normal, however, for a wife occasionally to place herself at the service of her husband if a special situation requires this submission. This fact alone does not make her action homosexual if she does not identify with him. The same behavior is not normal for a man. After all, there is a difference between the sexes, and this is one way in which it manifests itself.

Helping a woman enjoy sex or helping her reach climax is almost a socially accepted procedure in our culture. In part this must be explained by the current fear of the frustrated female, the monster who can, and sometimes does, devour her children and destroy her husband. But the fear of the female results only in further castration of the male and this in turn will lead to further frustration of the female. The man must be careful that in his desire for mutual pleasure and satisfaction, he does not surrender his own masculine identity nor accept a subservient role in the relationship. The 'good lover' is generally a poor male. Unfortunately, it seems to be part of the homosexual trend in our culture to equate masculine sexuality with the ability to satisfy a woman. But the woman is never truly satisfied with such a performance by the male, whether in the course of coital sex relations or in any other way. The so-called sex techniques end with the man losing more than he gains, with the woman losing what she truly wants—a man.

It is said that every homosexual is a latent heterosexual. Is the reverse true? Certainly latent homosexuality exists. It manifests itself in the behavior we discussed above and in dreams and fantasies. It manifests itself also in defense reactions against homosexuality, in the fear of and fascination with it. In a culture which places a premium on aggressiveness and virility, much vital energy is bound up in the defense against latent homosexual feelings. The male who carries himself as if he must impress one with his masculinity (broad shoulders, chest held up, stomach in, hard tight buttocks) is suspect of having latent homosexual attitudes. The man who is afraid of expressing or demonstrating any warmth or tenderness to another man by physical contact betrays a homosexual fear.

Depth analysis of patients has revealed the presence of latent homosexual tendencies in every case. By extension, since there are no perfectly healthy beings in our culture, homosexuality (latent or patent, to some degree or other) must be present in all individuals in our culture. This should be neither surprising nor shocking if one is at all aware of the sexual difficulties which people have. Study of these problems in patients permits us to state that homosexual tendencies exist in an individual to the degree that his sexual potency is disturbed or limited in the heterosexual sphere.

In our culture sexual behavior or attitudes can be ranged on a scale of potency with homosexuality at one end and heterosexuality at the other. This is a good working concept since it avoids the division of people into one class or the other. People are not heterosexuals or homosexuals, they are simply individuals with varying degrees of sexual potency. The more the potency, the more one tends to heterosexual patterns or sexuality; the less the potency, the more one manifests behavior that is characteristic of homosexuality.

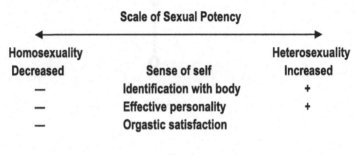

Scale of Sexual Potency

Homosexuality Decreased	Sense of self	Heterosexuality Increased
—	Identification with body	+
—	Effective personality	+
—	Orgastic satisfaction	

Fig. 4

The last item may require some explanation. The ability to achieve a satisfactory orgastic release is a function of sexual potency. Therefore it is limited to the heterosexual mode of functioning. Since the homosexual pattern is to derive pleasure and satisfaction through identification and acting out, the homosexual foregoes the experience of the self. And orgasm is nothing but self-experience or self-realization in its highest form.

There are important therapeutic implications from this analysis of homosexuality. If one can give a patient a better identification with his body, a stronger sense of self, a better functioning personality, the sexual pattern will automatically shift toward heterosexual behavior. Of course, to do this requires the working out of personality problems on one hand and body tensions on the other. However, the corollary is also true. Any increase in heterosexual feeling or behavior will lead to an improvement in all personality functions.

Finally we can say that the personality is a reflection of heterosexuality and vice versa. The diagram shown in the preceding lecture can be modified above.

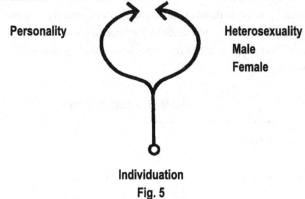

Personality   **Heterosexuality**
                         Male
                         Female

Individuation
Fig. 5

LECTURE III: THE NATURE OF THE ORGASTIC EXPERIENCE

Let us briefly review the points established in the preceding two lectures. In the first, we set forth the proposition that both sexuality and personality are products of the process of organismic development which we have called individuation. This means that, in the course of evolutionary history, as organisms developed increasing structure and complexity, their sexual characteristics became more sharply defined. At the same time, the unique individuality of each organism became more clearly evident.

Similarly, we find that in the growth and development of the individual person, the emerging personality is determined and conditioned by the strength and integration of the sexual drive. To support this proposition we attempted to show that sex and love are closely related—specifically, that sex is an expression of love, and that the feeling of love is a derivative of the sexual drive. This is important because the intimate connection between personality and love can hardly be denied.

We also attempted to show that the sex drive was brought into existence by the tendency of the living organism to produce excess energy which it must discharge. The discharge of this excess energy through the sexual mode of reproduction serves the function of maintaining the structure and integrity of the individual organism. Since the excess energy of the organism is the quantitative factor in personality, that is, since it measures the vitality of the organism, we can say that sexuality and personality are quantitatively equal.

In the second lecture, in discussing the difference between homosexuality and heterosexuality, we set forth our view that sexuality and personality are also equal on the qualitative level. The concept of a spectrum of sexual potency enabled us to postulate the identity of heterosexuality with (1) the development of the sense of self, or individuality; (2) a positive identification with the body; (3) an integrated and effective personality structure; and (4) orgastic potency. Homosexuality, which was placed at the opposite end of the scale, was correlated with the absence of these positive personality features, that is, with the lack of a sense of the self, an over-identification with the other, tendencies to act out either sadistic or masochistic patterns of behavior, and a personality geared to the idea of "service."

The concept of sexual potency has a two-fold aspect. It can refer on the one hand to the strength of the sexual desire or drive, and on the other to the intensity and totality of the sexual discharge. The latter is more properly called orgastic potency, which is the proper subject of this third lecture: the nature and subjective feeling of the orgastic experience.

Before we consider the question of orgasm, however, I think it is necessary to say a few words about the nature of pleasure. Important as this feeling is in the life and health of people, the nature and dynamics of pleasure are not discussed in any of the standard textbooks of physiology. In fact, pleasure as a motivating force in behavior is completely ignored by physiologists and biochemists. Only in analytic writing and thinking do we find any attempt to understand what pleasure is.

Freud propounded the idea that pleasure resulted from the discharge of tension. For example, one finds pleasure and satisfaction in hunger. Hunger represents a state of tension which is discharged in the process of its satisfaction or satisfied in the process of its discharge. If we consider the pleasure derived from the satisfactory evacuation of a bowel movement, we can see that it too derives from the discharge of a state of tension. Even the pleasure of achieving a difficult task can be related to the discharge of a tension which arose through the confrontation and challenge of the task.

The same principle holds true for sexual pleasure. The excess energy to which we have previously referred creates a state of tension which, when it is discharged through a satisfactory sexual experience, produces a significant pleasure experience.

But there is another sort of pleasure which does not fit into Freud's concept and which has not led to some modification of his theories.

According to Freud, pleasure results from discharge of tension. This has been interpreted as a statement that man strives for Nirvana, that is, for a state of no tension. Of course, this is not true. Many psychologists and analysts have pointed out that man often seeks out situations of stress and tension. Actually one can experience a certain amount of pleasure in the state of tension itself. This may be called "anticipatory pleasure." Thus there is pleasure in undertaking a challenging task as well as pleasure in completing the task. Similarly, the prospect of a good meal, even when one is in a state of hunger-tension, is experienced as pleasurable.

But the prospect of a challenging situation can be pleasurable provided that one can anticipate the satisfactory resolution of the tension situation. The pleasure in a state of tension depends upon the existence in the mind of the person of the prospect of releasing the tension. Take the prospect away and every state of tension or of excitation would become unpleasurable and frustrating. In fact, frustration is nothing but a state of excitation or tension from which there is no prospect of release. Given the prospect of release, we can tolerate the tension until the possibility of its discharge occurs.

Pleasure has a dual nature like sexual potency. First there is the pleasure of the excitation, provided that one can anticipate its discharge, and then there is the pleasure of the release of the tension or the discharge of the excitation. In terms of excitation, this can be expressed as the pleasure of the increase in the excitation, anticipation, and the pleasure of the discharge of the excitation, satisfaction.

Seen in this light, pleasure is not the experience of a static state but of a dynamic one. The organism does not seek to discharge tension as an end in itself, nor does it seek to build tension as an end in itself. If a state of excitation were not discharged, the organism could not get excited again. Rather, if it seeks anything, it seeks the movement from one state to another.

Movement is perhaps the most basic function in the living organism. The organism is alive because it moves and it moves because it is alive. Its pleasure derives from its movements, both towards the world and away from the world. Frustration is the inability to move out of a state of excitation. Depression is the inability to move into a state of excitation.

We have indicated that movement is produced by the increase and decrease of excitation in the organism. An increase moves the organism toward the exciting object, while a decrease of excitation moves it away from the object. To understand the orgastic experience, it is important to know the goal of sexual activity is not the presence or absence of a state of tension but the process of increase and decrease in the state of excitation. The result is a quickened movement and a greater sense of aliveness, both of which are experienced as pleasurable by the organism. Movement, aliveness and pleasure all contribute to a heightened perception of the self. The dual nature of pleasure can be shown graphically:

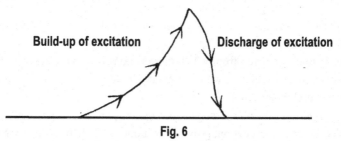

Build-up of excitation   **Discharge of excitation**

Fig. 6

Let us see how these concepts apply to the sexual function. First we must stress that the sexual drive depends upon the existence of excess energy in the organism, that is, upon the availability of energy over and beyond that needed to maintain biological survival. Since the production of excess energy is a natural function of living, its quantity is a measure of aliveness or vitality. The corollary is evident. There is no sex drive in dead persons nor can one be aroused no matter what stimuli are applied. Anything which depletes the energy of the organism reduces the sexual drive. Illness, fatigue, lack of sleep and neurotic tensions are among the causes which act in this direction. The factors which act in the opposite direction are those which promote the natural health and vitality of the organism. I know of no artificial stimulants to the sexual drive. Alcohol may increase the desire, but it decreases the function.

This excess energy is diffused through the organism. Or it may be said to exist as a state of latent excitation. In the normal course of events, either with or without external stimulation, this energy will flow toward its natural outlet, which is the genital apparatus. Once the energy becomes focused upon the genitals, we become conscious of the feeling of sexual arousal. Arousal is not a process of putting feeling or life into a person; the general feeling or life must be there first. Arousal is a result of focus. This focus upon the genital apparatus can develop spontaneously or through an outer stimulus if the individual has available some excess energy, some latent excitation, or a generalized feeling of well-being.

Once focus occurs, any contact or further contact with a member of the opposite sex will operate to increase the focus, that is, raise the level of sexual excitation and further the urge for sexual union. This is the function of those activities which we describe as forepleasure.

Forepleasure serves two purposes relative to the sexual function: (1) to mobilize through the contact of the bodies the available excess energy normally locked in different parts of the body; and (2) to increase the level of excitation. Energy is mobilized from the mouth or oral zones, from the breast, the neck and the back, the skin, etc., and focused upon the genital organs. As this happens the excitatory state of the organism is increased so that a greater urgency is felt for sexual union and sexual discharge. The build-up of sexual excitation through forepleasure mechanisms is experienced pleasurably as a life-positive force as long as it is possible to anticipate the release of the tension.

The second phase of sexual activity embraces those actions which lead to sexual discharge. These constitute end-pleasure mechanisms, the goal of which is not to heighten the tension but to release it. The pleasure of the discharge differs from the pleasure of the excitation. This difference can only be described as the feeling of fulfillment and satisfaction as opposed to excitation and anticipation.

The end-pleasure of discharge can be only as intense as the excitation which preceded it. However, I do not wish to give the impression that the sexual act can be easily divided into arbitrary periods. The process of excitation continues through the act of coitus until the involuntary movements of discharge occur. Thus one can enter into a sexual relation without a high degree of conscious excitation and realize, nevertheless, a strong and satisfactory climax. In this case, excitation mounts in the act of intercourse. The voluntary sexual movements create considerable excitement in addition to the excitation of sexual contact.

No aspect of sexuality is more confused or misunderstood than the phenomenon of the orgasm. The term itself is used in two different senses which should be distinguished from each other. Commonly, the term is used as synonymous with climax; every climax is called an orgasm. In the other sense, the one used by W. Reich, orgasm is limited to the kind of climax or release which is total, fulfilling and completely satisfying. A climax is not an orgasm according to this meaning unless it reaches the acme of pleasure. Implied in the view of the concept of orgasm as ecstasy, the supreme culmination of desire, total fulfillment.

To avoid the confusion inherent in two opposing concepts, we should recognize that the orgastic experience can vary from any feeling of climax to the sublime realization of the self. The orgasm varies among individuals, depending upon their personality structure, as we shall see, but it also varies in the same individual according to the intensity of the sexual response in any particular sexual relation.

Before we go deeper into the nature of the orgasm, it would be interesting to know why Reich formulated a dynamic concept of orgastic potency. In his attempt to understand the factors which determined the success or failure of analytic therapy, Reich made two discoveries. First, he found that only to the degree that the patient's sexual function improved as a result of therapy was he able to hold on to and develop the fruits of the therapy. Second, he found a positive correlation between neurotic disturbance and the lack of sexual fulfillment. This meant that there could be no neurosis in the presence of a fully satisfactory sexual life. The analysts' response to this view was that they had many neurotic patients who were capable of experiencing sexual satisfaction. This contradiction necessitated a definition of "satisfaction" in sex. It became evident to Reich that the analysts equated climax with total fulfillment. Between the two there may be a world of difference.

The orgasm, as Reich defined it and as we will use it in this lecture, presupposes a total involuntary pleasurable discharge of all the excess energy of the organism. By excess energy we mean energy that is not immediately needed for the maintenance of basic biological functions. If this happens, then theoretically there would be no energy left to support a neurotic symptom or a neurotic character structure. The neurotic symptom would collapse as the energy needed to maintain it is drained away in the orgastic discharge.

Now this can and does happen. When a person achieves orgastic potency in the sense of a total bodily and personality response in sex, he becomes free of his neurotic symptoms for as long as he can maintain that level of sexual functioning. Unfortunately, neurotic habits are very deeply ingrained in the personality and without their resolution analytically, the old pattern reasserts itself and undermines the sexual function. The reason for this is that the neurotic pattern determines behavior in all activities and in all relationships. Faced with the vicissitudes of everyday living, the neurotic falls back on his defenses and compensations.

It becomes necessary, therefore, to work out the neurotic problems on two levels. On the level of personality, the neurosis must be analyzed according to character-analytic procedures. But the sexual function must be improved in the course of this work. Without a dynamic concept of orgastic potency as a guide to the sexual function, one is at a loss to know why patients fail to show the progress which their intellectual insight seems to warrant.

With this preliminary explanation over, we may ask: what is the nature of this phenomenon (orgasm) which makes it so imperative an urge for all living creatures? How can it function to discharge all the excess energy of the organism?

Reich had shown that the orgasm occurs as a convulsive reaction in which the total body participates, a reaction which he called the orgasm-reflex. This reaction takes the form of a series of involuntary pelvic movements which embrace the total body in a succession of waves moving upward from below. To understand these movements we must know something about the mechanics of energy flow in the organism. Specifically, it is important to understand why the sexual function is located at the tail end of the organism.

To explain my views, I should like to use the fish as an example. The drawing is not intended as a work of art.

The fish is interesting because while it literally moves through its environment, the environment moves through the fish. Not only does the fish go through the water, but the water goes through the fish—a two-way interaction. The head end of the fish is where the environment enters the fish: water, food, sense impressions. At the head end are located the functions which take in or charge the organism. At the tail end, discharge occurs in the form of elimination, sexual discharge and movement. The fish shows a polarity in its dynamic function. As it moves forward, energy is moving backward through its body to be discharged in the movement of the tail. The movements of the sexual act and of the orgasm are also movements of the tail or tail end of the organism.

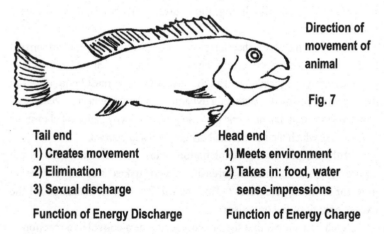

Direction of movement of animal

Fig. 7

Tail end	Head end
1) Creates movement	1) Meets environment
2) Elimination	2) Takes in: food, water
3) Sexual discharge	sense-impressions
Function of Energy Discharge	**Function of Energy Charge**

The fish moving through its liquid environment is an isolated individual. No matter how much it may feel part of its surroundings, the fact of its individuality is biologically determined by the fact that it is a closed system. Its motility is dependent upon a free energy contained within an enclosed body. We have previously suggested that every animal organism needs to give up its individuality, to overcome its sense of aloneness and apartness, to become part of the whole which is also experienced as self-completion. We suggested also that it accomplishes this through sexuality by means of which it joins with another organism and loses its sense of aloneness and incompleteness. But more than this is involved. The very quality of its movements which are inherent in individuality has to change. It has to move in a different way, a mode of movement which is a part of a larger movement, a movement that goes back to its origin and creation.

One can overcome the sense of aloneness and incompleteness by certain passive procedures. Meditation, religious isolation and self-communion, mysticism are some of the methods employed. Passivity, however, is not the natural way of life. By union with another organism, an excitation is set up which is capable of moving the organism. In the feeling of being moved, we experience ourselves as part of the universal. Precisely because religion can move us (in the emotional sense) do we experience it as a valid expression of our link with God. Sexual intercourse does this in a direct and physical way.

The following statement is one woman's experience of this phenomenon. Her description is concise and revealing.

> Once I had an experience during intercourse which was so different from anything else that I don't think I will ever be satisfied until I experience it again. During this experience, without any effort or trying on my part, my body was moved from within, so to speak, and everything was right. There was rhythmic movement and a feeling of ecstasy at being part of something much greater than myself, and finally of reward, of real satisfaction and peace.

Let me illustrate this process of union and movement with a set of simplified drawings.

(a)

Two animals approach each other.

(b)

Assuming that there is an attraction between them, they will line up.

(c)

Line-up is followed by what Reich called super-imposition. The dominant animal mounts the other. The male generally mounts the female and penetrates.

(d)

As a result of the sexual movements, both voluntary and involuntary, a spin is created.

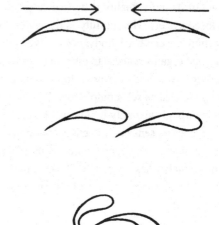

Fig. 8

At the moment of spin, male and female are no longer distinguishable. The energy streams of the two organisms become one spinning process. When the phenomenon of spinning is free and uninhibited, in the sexual climax or orgasm, the result is an experience of lumination or glow in the two organisms. The glow sets in first in the pelvis about the genital organs as a higher stage of the "heat" of sexual passion. Depending upon the intensity and extent of the orgastic feeling the glow can extend over the whole body when it is experienced as a lumination. The external manifestation of the lumination is seen as a radiance which is the natural expression of a person in love.

When one looks at the diagram in **d**, one may note its resemblance to the spinning of spiral nebulae. This resemblance was pointed out by Reich as an illustration of man's roots in nature. It is in this phenomenon of spinning and glow that the individual experiences cosmic identification in orgasm. The sensations experienced in orgasm are also frequently described as feelings of flying or whirling. In one of his novels, Hemingway described orgasm as the feeling that "the earth moved." Orgasm fulfills the longing of the animal to get beyond the limits of the self, to transcend the narrow confines of individuality.

The movement in orgasm differs from the normal movements in a significant way. Normal movements are ego-directed, that is, they are produced by the flow of excitation from head to tail end. In orgasm, something takes possession of the body. The excitation flows from tail end to the head. It is as if the normal pattern of dog-wags-tail is reversed, so that now the tail wags the dog. There is a loss of ego in the orgasm as some deeper life force takes over. The self, not the ego, is realized on its deepest level.

The orgastic experience has other meanings. It is experienced as a rebirth, a renewal. This finds some explanation in the feelings of melting and flow which precede the orgastic convulsion. Since the structure of the body is composed in part of crystalline water (even at normal body temperature, as current research shows), the melting and flowing sensations may be interpreted as the thawing out of these crystalline water structures. Structure, being the opposite of motility, is the antithesis of life. Life begins with very little structure and ends when the energy of the organism is incapable of moving the accumulated structures which the experience of living creates. So when structure is dissolved in orgasm, we are truly being reborn as our perception of the experience tells us. Orgasm is also experienced as a creative phenomenon. Sometimes it actually results in the creation of a new individual. But at all times it results in the creation of a new and fresh vision of life.

If sexuality is oriented toward the satisfaction and fulfillment of orgastic discharge, sensuality is aimed at increasing the state of sexual excitement. Normally, sensuality is part of the sexual process. The simulation of all the senses plays an important role in the preliminary phase of sexual excitation. It aids in mobilizing the excess energy of the organism, it increases the focus upon the genital apparatus, and it heightens the excitatory state. Forepleasure is a predominantly sensual experience. But sensuality can become opposed to sexuality if the search for excitation becomes an end in itself. The sensualist differs from the sexual person in that he is less interested in the end-pleasure of discharge than he is in the excitation of forepleasure and stimulation.

What factors in the personality of the individual dispose him to a sensual approach to life rather than a sexual one? Clinical experience has shown that a sensual attitude is determined by two traits in the personality make-up. One is a lack of excess energy or aliveness; the other is fear of the sexual climax—the orgasm. Let us analyze each of these.

The search for excitation characterizes persons who are unalive, depressed, morally and physically debilitated. Lacking an inner feeling of excitement, they feel that life is boring. Sex, like any other strong stimulant, gives them a temporary feeling of excitement or aliveness. They use sex like an alcoholic uses drink. Since the stimulation is only temporary, the pursuit of excitation is pushed to greater lengths. Forepleasure is extended to a degree where it becomes a perversion, as Freud pointed out. If this is not enough, the sensualist seeks excitement by creating external situations of tension. He engages in sexual activity in exposed places or in the presence of third persons. The sexual act is performed before mirrors so that the visual excitement can increase the feeling. Special techniques to arouse the partner are employed so that he can gain some vicarious excitement through the reaction of his partner.

Now, I am not a sexual moralist and my intent is not to condemn these practices. The sensualist needs such practices to gain sufficient excitement to make some sexual function possible. He needs sexuality as we all do to overcome his isolation and loneliness. But the immoderate use of sensuality, like alcohol, ends in disappointment and a feeling of hangover. The sensualist wakes up the next day with no feeling of cleanness, no feeling of fulfillment, no feeling of renewal or rebirth.

And his activity has been of no help in overcoming his characterological condition of deadness and boredom.

The second reason for the sensual attitude is fear of orgastic discharge with its strong, involuntary and convulsive movements. Reich called this fear 'orgasm-anxiety.' It may seem strange that one should be afraid of pleasure, but pleasure-anxiety is typical of all neurotic persons. Pleasure, especially sexual pleasure, is associated on the conscious or unconscious level with sin and guilt. While sexual guilt has diminished considerably since Victorian times, it has by no means been eliminated. Beneath the surface of our present-day sexual sophistication one can find deep layers of sexual guilt in most individuals. For reasons which will be apparent soon, this guilt is attached to orgastic sexuality more than to sensual sexuality. It is my experience that our sexual sophistication has lowered the barriers to sensuality without significantly affecting or relieving orgasm-anxiety. To appreciate this anomaly, we must fully understand the movements which lead to sexual orgasm.

The normal waking movements of the individual are ego-directed and ego-controlled. Our activities are purposeful and goal-directed. The average person walks to get to a destination. When one observes people walking, however, one is often impressed with the mechanical quality of the movement. Both in ourselves and others we sense the lack of pleasure in walking; we are aware only of the urgency to get somewhere. Of course, as soon as one goal is reached, another is envisaged. On the cultural level this is exemplified in our concept of progress. The pleasure of movement, the joy in the coordination and gracefulness of motion is missing from our normal daily activities. We have become so ego-conscious that we have lost consciousness of the self represented by the body in motion. But to this extent we do not have strong and secure ego-structures.

Less civilized people show a different quality in their body movements. When one watches a West Indian woman walk, for example, one is aware of the ease and freedom of the body. The hips sway loosely, the legs move effortlessly, while the upper half of the body rides gracefully upon this carriage. The native woman is not pressed to arrive anywhere on time.

The Voice of the Body

But what strikes us most about this kind of walking is its sexual quality. It is sexual, not because it is provocative, but because it looks vital, alive, animal-like. It is sexual because the woman is conscious of her movements and is identified with the sexual nature of her body.

Sexuality is our strongest link with our animal natures. The animal knows no goals other than the satisfaction of his immediate needs. He labors under no compulsion to progress. He finds his pleasure in the activity of the moment. What is the goal of sexuality other than the pleasure of sexuality? One "goes" nowhere with the sexual movements. In sexuality one allows the movements to direct the person, not the reverse. It is like a dog following his nose, not directing it. Watching a dog lope along, one has the impression that his body moves him, he does not move his body. This ability of the body to move the person is the capacity to have orgastic experience.

Orgastic potency represents the ability to let the body take over the movement. But one cannot permit this to happen unless one is secure in the body and identified with it. If the body is subordinate to the ego on one hand, it is in relationship to the ground, on the other. The latter relationship provides the feeling of being grounded and furnishes the security for the loss of ego control in orgastic climax. To feel grounded also means to be rooted in the earth and in sexuality. It is synonymous with the ability to stand on your own feet (be independent) and to feel them, to be identified with the lower half of the body in its basic animal functions.

We have said that the sexual movement differs from normal movements in its direction. It is a movement from the ground upward rather than a movement from the head downward. But this distinction is not fully valid, for to some extent all movement should partake of this sexual quality. In the healthy person, movement will show a dual relationship, animal-like, sexual and grounded below while poised, goal-directed and controlled above. Sexuality is not a part-time or leisure activity; it is a way of functioning. Sexuality means being in contact with the ground and the body at the same time that one is in contact with the mind and the external world. Sexuality means being a thinking person and a moving animal organism at the same time.

Emotional health represents the ability to be in two places at once, that is, it means one has the strength to tolerate the tension of a polar situation. As I stand before you lecturing, I have to be aware of you and aware of myself. I have to be in touch with you and in touch with myself. Yet a moment's introspection will show that that one cannot be in two places at the same time. However, it is possible to oscillate the attention so rapidly that there is no perceptible break in the dual awareness. Thus, for a moment I turn back to myself while lecturing, look at my notes and feel myself, then I turn to you. If it is done smoothly, you are not aware of any break in my contact with you and I am not aware of a break in my contact with myself.

Similarly, one can be in contact with the body and the ground and in contact with the thinking and sensing self, not simultaneously, but alternately, and yet with such rapidity of oscillation that one is aware of both. If these experiences are part of one's way of life, then the transition from ego-control and voluntary movement to the strong involuntary movements of orgasm becomes easier and not frightening. Otherwise orgasm becomes equal to the threat of being whirled into space at the end of a rocket.

Reich, in *The Function of the Orgasm*, set forth what in his opinion was the curve of sexual excitation and orgasm. This curve is set forth below as a basis for our further discussion of this subject.

As we said earlier in this lecture, one can designate any climax as an orgasm or one can restrict the term *orgasm* to the meaning used by Reich. Only the latter meaning enables us to understand the varied disturbances in sexual potency.

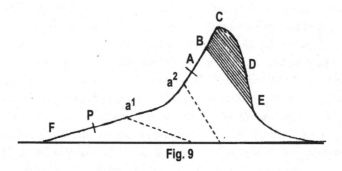

Fig. 9

F – Period of forepleasure

P – Penetration

A – Increase in frequency of pelvic movements, becoming involuntary; strong melting sensations in pelvis.

B – Convulsive body movements

C – Climax or acme

D – Sharp decline in excitation, flow back to body

R – Relaxation

BCDE – Shaded area represents the orgastic experience. At E the involuntary movements stop.

a^1 – Climax in the case of premature ejaculation. The excitation subsides gradually. There is no feeling of release or fulfillment. The clitoral climax in a woman has a similar quality.

a^2 – Climax where discharge occurs before the involuntary movements have taken over. A climax occurring at this point reveals fear of the involvement phase of sexual movement.

During the phase from P to A, the sexual movements are under ego-control. The movements are slow, gentle and relaxed. They may be interrupted to allow for adjustment of position or for short periods of rest. Interruption at this time does not interfere with the course of the excitation. Generally the movements of the man and woman are not synchronized at this phase. This is slowly achieved in the course of feeling each other's passion. The voluntary movements also serve to unify the body with the movements so that the rhythm of breathing and thrust become one. Gradually the direction of the movement shifts so that the forward thrust is made more and more from the ground or the feet.

At A the tempo of the sexual movements increases. This is a voluntary act by the male, done after he feels that his partner's movements have become synchronized with his own and that both are ready for the ascent to the climax. In the course of the increasing tempo, the movements suddenly become involuntary. At the end of this phase strong melting sensations appear in the pelvis preliminary to the beginning of discharge.

At B the total body participates in the convulsive reaction. Excitement still mounts for the man as ejaculation begins, and remains at a high peak for a few moments. During the phase B to C to D, the organism may be described as 'spinning.' It is during this period that the sensations of cosmic identification and lumination are experienced.

At D the excitation begins to subside rapidly as energy and feeling flow back into the body. The involuntary movements persist until E, when relaxation, frequently leading to the desire for sleep, takes over.

Pleasure is experienced both in the course of the increase and in the course of the decrease of excitation. The former, however, has an anticipatory quality. The latter yields satisfaction if the discharge of tension is total, that is, if all the excess energy of the organism is mobilized into the sexual feeling. In both a^1 and a^2 the inability to reach the acme at C means that a total mobilization has not occurred. Neither in a^1 nor a^2 is there a true feeling of satisfaction. Further, the intensity of the experience of pleasure is a function of the change in level of excitation during a given period of time. The greater the amount of excitation or tension discharged within a unit of time, the greater the pleasure. In a^2 the level of tension or excitation falls off gradually. Very little pleasure is felt. In a^2, where the tension is discharged more rapidly, the experience is more pleasurable.

Any discharge which occurs after B is both intensely pleasurable and satisfying.

What determines the ability of an individual to have an orgasm of the kind described? We have indicated some of the attributes earlier. We remarked that a person must be grounded, which is merely another way of saying that he must feel secure in himself. We added that he must stand on his own feet, which means that he must be independent. Without these qualities, he cannot move in a sexual way, that is, from the ground. But we can also say that he must be identified with his body in its sexual nature and free from any sexual guilt or inhibition. These attributes may be expressed in three words: security, independence, and pride.

The individual who possesses these attributes would necessarily have a strong and well-developed ego. His ego-structure would parallel and reflect his strong sexual feelings. And he would need a strong ego-structure to tolerate and sustain the building-up of tension and excitation as the sexual movements gain increasing frequency and intensity and tend to become involuntary. Neurotic individuals with weak and underdeveloped egos could not sustain the tension necessary to reach the heights where orgasm occurs. If, therefore, the ego is overwhelmed in the orgastic discharge, it presupposes that one has an ego to be overwhelmed. To lose a self, one must have a self. But only if one loses one's self does one gain a self.

Certain physical attributes are required if one is to experience orgasm. The individual must be an alive and vital person. One must have an excess of energy if the sexual excitation is to be significantly experienced. The body should show a harmony of its parts; it should have a feeling of unity about its movements which should be graceful and coordinated. If this seems too much to ask, please remember that orgasm is the result of a unitary movement in the body from below upward. But this would not be possible if unity was absent from the normal movements of the body. All that we are saying is an elaboration of the theme of sex and personality. Orgasm, which is the highest form of sexual response, characterizes the sexual behavior of the mature, integrated and effective personality.

We can reach the same conclusions from the very nature of the orgasm as a satisfactory experience. Satisfaction in any activity can be obtained only if one commits one's entire energy to the activity. Anything less than a total commitment cannot provide a physical feeling of satisfaction. This is true whether one plays a game, undertakes a work project or engages in sex. Win or lose, having committed yourself totally, you will feel satisfied with your effort.

What is total commitment in sex? Certainly any division of attention, like smoking a cigarette or reading a book while having sex relations is an obvious lack of commitment. Sexual fantasies indicate an inability to make a full commitment to the sexual partner. But the holding back can be unconscious. Therefore a total commitment can be gauged only by the totality and unity of the sexual movement. Only if the sexual movement embraces the total body or being will one experience the full satisfaction of orgastic discharge.

But the orgastic experience can vary even in the same person. If satisfaction depends upon the extent of involvement or commitment, the intensity of the orgasm must depend upon the depth of feelings involved. In its deepest depths, the sexual response actively involves the heart. When the heart responds in the sexual climax, the deepest and fullest feeling of opening up and release has been achieved. This feeling is experienced in the very center of one's being, that is, in the heart. Then one knows the deepest meaning of love.

In the first lecture we spoke of the relation of sex to love. In analyzing that relationship we pointed to the connection between the heart and the genitals via the blood. Sex was viewed as an expression of love. And so it is, but only to the degree that the individual experiences pleasure and satisfaction in sex. That is, if sex is an expression of love, as I believe, it expresses that love most fully in the response of orgasm.

We have used the term *satisfaction* to describe the pleasure of the orgastic experience. Satisfactory it truly is, but this term seems inadequate to indicate the true nature of this pleasure. This orgasm is not only pleasurable, it is a joyful experience. It is joyful because it is free, unrestrained, unlimited, and involuntary. It has the same quality as the emotional reactions of children: it comes from the heart. For that reason it is the highest expression of joy available to adults.

If the activities of the sensualist are marked by the search for excitement and fun, the truly sexual person is characterized by his joyfulness.

LECTURE IV: MALE AND FEMALE SEXUALITY

The remarks which I shall offer here about men and women should be taken as the expression of my personal opinions and judgments. These derive, of course, from seventeen years of clinical experience as a psychiatrist and therapist, from more than twenty years of study in the field of sexology and from my personal observations.

Unfortunately, there is no objectively scientific way to measure sexual responsivity so no one else has a better vantage point. Another qualification which I must make is that my statements are not to be taken as absolutes but rather as broad generalizations. They cannot be applied to the individual case without some modifications to allow for the personality differences of individuals. Nevertheless, they are valid as guideposts in the unknown and complex terrain of male and female sexuality.

An old story, which I am sure is familiar to you, is told of a convention of professional women who emphasized female accomplishments in many fields and concluded there was very little difference between the sexes. A drunken spectator cried, "Hooray for the difference." A French version ends with the declaration, "Vive la difference."

The nature of this difference poses a problem, a very important problem, for the relations of men and women. Some time ago *Look* featured on its cover the picture of a large woman with her foot upon a small prostrate man. The implication of this picture was that women in our culture have become the dominant sex. There are statistics to prove that in this country women own more property and wealth than men. Another indication of the changing relation between men and women is given by movies and television shows. Fairly often the man is pictured as stupid, blundering, egotistical and inferior to the woman in wisdom and understanding of life. I can refer you to the popular television show, "The Flintstones" as an example of this view. You may have seen the picture, "Mr. Hobbs Takes a Vacation, " which is another illustration of this attitude. Despite the fact that Mr. Hobbs is a successful executive, he is portrayed as a second class member of the family. His needs and pleasure are subservient to those of the other members of the family. He does all the chores and dirty work. His wife is always right with her counsel and advice, whereas he is invariably wrong. Yet after the vacation ends, which for Mr. Hobbs was somewhat of a fiasco, he remarks, "We'll have to go back and do it again next year." In one show after another the woman is portrayed as the one who knows the answers, makes the right remarks and knows more in contrast to her well-meaning, good-intentioned, but insensitive partner.

Perhaps the differences between the sexes are diminishing. One has the impression that women are becoming more masculine while men are becoming more feminine. Passive feminine attitudes in men do seem to be on the increase. The apparent increase in homosexuality bears this out. That it is common knowledge is shown by this popular joke: "Do you know why women try so hard to keep their girlish figures? To retain their boyish husbands."

At the same time one hears the constant complaint from women that the average male is not aggressive enough. In one of our local newspapers recently there was an article entitled, "The Trouble with Women is Men." This idea is frequently expressed by women in the observation that one man makes them feel like a woman while another does not. If it is true the other way around, and I have seen many castrating females, the man is generally not the one to complain. He assumes the responsibility for the success or failure of the relationship without knowing how or why it failed.

I believe we must face the fact that there is confusion and concern about the social and sexual roles of the man and woman in our present cultural situation. On one hand, the woman wants to be equal with the man in all things; on the other, she wants him to be the dominant figure. Men try to satisfy the needs of women only to find the latter unfulfilled and critical.

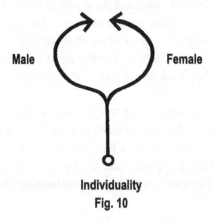

Male   **Female**

Individuality
Fig. 10

If a man dominates the home, he is considered dictatorial; if he is passive and submissive, he becomes inadequate. Now I cannot tell you how to walk this tightrope. I have never figured it out for myself. I think, however, that we can gain some understanding of male and female roles, sexually and socially, from an analysis of the biological factors involved in male and female sexuality. Our point of departure will be the dialectic proposition that individuality creates the antithesis of male and female. This is shown in the diagram. This diagram suggests that while man and woman are equal as individuals, they are opposite to each other or antithetically related in terms of sexual function. This means that on one level there are similarities, while on another there are significant differences.

Let us consider first the sexual similarities between man and woman. We know that women are similar to men in their basic biological functions. They eat, sleep, defecate exactly as a man does; they respond to the same sedation and they are excited by the same stimulants. Bioenergetically, their organisms become charged with energy or excitation which seeks discharge just like the man's organism. Pleasure and satisfaction in sex are as important to a woman as they are to a man. More specifically, the orgasm as we described it in the previous lecture is experienced in identical fashion by the man and the woman. Thus, the woman as well as the man can experience the sensation of spinning or flying, the sense of cosmic identification, the feeling of ecstasy, the feeling of release with loss of the boundaries or limitations of ego and personality and the glow of radiance which accompany the full orgastic discharge of the excitation.

The pelvic movements in the woman parallel those in the man. There are some differences in rhythm in the first stages of coitus but these become ironed out into a harmonic movement, as the excitation builds to its climax. At the acme the involuntary movements are so matched that one loses the awareness of the boundary between one's self and the partner.

The woman's sexual responsivity depends on the same factors which determine sexual potency in the male: the aliveness and vitality of her organism, her identification with her body, the coordination of her movements; that is, her sexual potency depends on the integrity and development of her ego and her personality. This view of female sexuality is supported by the research of Reich as well as by my own observations.

I have said that the course of excitation, in terms of the build-up and release of tension, is identical in the woman and in the man. This statement must be modified in those cases where cultural or neurotic factors have disturbed the normal sexual rhythms. These disturbances are so common that they have given rise to the myth that the woman is slower to sexual arousal and to climax than the man. In a culture whose sexual patterns encourage sexual passivity on the part of the woman, we can anticipate some disturbance of natural response. Certainly, the operation of a "double standard" of sexual behavior for the man and for the woman will interfere with the natural rhythm of sexual response.

There is a strange effect of neurotic disturbances upon male and female sexuality which points to differences which we shall consider later. One effect of neurosis upon the male is to create the condition of premature ejaculation. This happens because the tensions in the pelvic area associated with the neurosis make it difficult for the man to tolerate the strong melting sensations which precede and accompany the full orgasm. In a woman the same neurotic problem acts to delay or slow down the build-up of her excitation. The result is that while the neurotic woman generally takes longer to reach a climax, the neurotic man comes quicker. The effect is that they are unable to "come" together and this must be taken literally. Physical closeness and intimacy which is a major objective of sexual activity is denied the neurotic individual. He cannot have it because he is afraid of it, which is merely another way of saying that he has a neurotic problem.

There is another myth going around which says that simultaneous orgasms are neither important to sexual pleasure nor particularly desirable. This view of sexuality would encourage one party to satisfy the other, who would then return the service. I expressed my opinion about this form of sexual behavior in the lecture on homosexual versus heterosexual attitudes, in sex. If spontaneous, simultaneous orgasm has become a myth, it is like the myth of freedom in communist countries. If people have lived without freedom for more than a generation, it becomes difficult to remember when it existed or what it was like. And the newer generation would have more trouble with the concept of freedom than the older. Freedom would become a myth as George Orwell points out in his story, "The Animal Farm." Well, a similar thing has happened with respect to sexuality. There has been such a loss of sexual potency in our time that joy, ecstasy and simultaneity of orgasm seem almost to be a myth.

The problem of the neurotic gap between male and female sexual responsiveness is responsible for the advocacy of special techniques in sex. The man can attempt to overcome this gap in several ways. He can try to inhibit the build-up of excitation and delay his climax until the woman is ready to reach her climax. This maneuver generally defeats itself since the exercise of control by the man inhibits the feeling of passion which is of the essence in the relationship. A woman's sexual response depends in part at least on the man's state of excitation. He can try to stimulate the woman before penetration so that she will be in a greater state of readiness once coitus is undertaken. However, if forepleasure activities are prolonged, end pleasure or orgasm suffers. A woman is physiologically ready as soon as she is moist and lubricated. A third means which is commonly employed to cope with this problem is the manual stimulation of the woman's clitoris during intercourse by the man. Every man to whom I have spoken who has engaged in this practice has resented it. The woman gains so little from it that it is not worth the trouble. My recommendation that it be discontinued has proved to be a relief to both parties.

It is in the very nature of this problem that all techniques must fail. There seems to be no other way for these specific disturbances to be eliminated than by the working through of the neurotic problems which cause them. In other words, only by the man becoming more secure in his manhood and the woman more identified with her feminine nature can a way be found for human beings to overcome their sexual frustration and achieve sexual happiness.

Though it is beyond the scope of this lecture, a word should be said about the difference between the vaginal orgasm and a clitoral orgasm. In the sense in which we have used the term *orgasm* earlier, the clitoral orgasm is not a true orgasm. It does not yield any of the sensations or feelings which we have said characterize the orgastic experience. However, it is a climax and does produce some feeling of release. Let me illustrate the difference by quoting the observations of the woman.

The vaginal orgasm feels right. I know this is the way it should be. It involves my whole pelvis and sometimes my legs. The clitoral orgasm is on the surface and there is very little feeling in the vagina. The muscles of my thighs remain very tense after a clitoral orgasm. After a vaginal orgasm, I feel relaxed and fulfilled.

Here is another comment:

The vaginal orgasms I've experienced, limited as they may have been, filled me with a sense of completeness, of satisfaction, a feeling of being full—filled up. The clitoral orgasm is more high level in excitement, but leaves no after effect of completion. I feel I could have another one right away.

The consensus is that the clitoral orgasm is superficial and unfulfilling. Only the vaginal orgasm results in complete relaxation. To understand this difference, we must know something about the development of sexuality in man and woman. The simplified schematic presentation below illustrates three stages in this development.

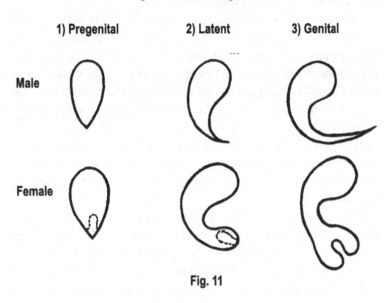

Fig. 11

The pregenital period from birth to about 3 to 4 years of age is characterized by the progressive integration of the pregenital libidinal zones or partial impulses into a coordinated individual in whom genital reality functions have become anchored at both ends of the orgasm, at the head and in the ego and below in genitality. During this period the main emphasis is upon the fulfillment of the organism's oral needs: security, affection, attention, and food. These constitute, in a psychological sense, narcissistic supplies which are necessary to the development of the individuality of the growing child. In this stage the child discovers its body; that is, it develops a body image based upon a unified sense of perception and a unitary and coordinated motor response.

In this stage there is no functional difference between male and female. The differences are there but they are not functional. There is little in the behavior of a boy or girl child even at four years of age to indicate its sex. The young child functions primarily as an undifferentiated individual. The attitude of the parents toward the young child should be one of *respect* for its developing individuality.

From about 4 or 5 years of age to puberty the child passes through a stage which is known in analytic literature as the latent period. The latent period is characterized by the child's growing awareness of its genitals and recognition of its role as a boy or girl. The child is aware only of superficial differences, that is, of the peripheral structures. The boy knows that he has a penis, the girl that she has an opening. The vagina is closed off by the hymen as the glans is enclosed and protected by the foreskin, assuming that circumcision has not been done. I believe that circumcision is detrimental to the developing sexuality of the boy. The foreskin is not to be interfered with any more than the hymen is to be broken.

The masturbation of a boy or girl in this stage shows little awareness of the mature sexual functions which lie dormant within except in those cases where the child has become the object of adult sexual feelings. In masturbation, both explore the genital area. There is an overall feeling of excitement but no strong focus of feelings on the genitals occurs. Neither attempts to masturbate to climax or satisfaction. The masturbation of the girl is not specific. There is no distinction between clitoris and vagina. She experiences pleasure in manual contact with the genital area and a feeling of the totality of her physical being. The body image is almost completed in this period. The feelings and sensations which underlie the body image provide the physical basis for the emerging personality which becomes shaped in this period. The latent period is devoted to the child's personality, which bursts into bloom with the eruption of mature genitality.

Proper upbringing demands respect on the part of the parents for the developing personality of the child. The boy is treated with respect for his oncoming manhood as the girl is to be respected for her forthcoming womanhood.

The third stage is designated as the genital stage. It can be further subdivided into adolescence, the late teens, and sexual maturity. For purposes of brevity we shall avoid these possible distinctions. Let us follow the biological development.

In the boy the development continues along the same line it had previously followed. The genital feeling becomes stronger and is experienced as an outward drive represented by the erection of the penis. In the course of these early erections the foreskin is stretched and the head is protruded. Sexual masturbation also involves the activation of the mechanism of ejaculation and the production of mature sperm cells. On the chart this is indicated by the extension of the point. Bioenergetically, the penis may be considered to be an extension of the coccyx or tail bone. This concept is derived from the masculine pelvic thrust which is experienced as a feeling flowing down the back, around the pelvis and into the penis.

In the girl marked changes occur at puberty in contrast to the boy whose development proceeds in a straight direction. The pelvis enlarges disproportionately and tilts backward. The vagina which in a girl is in a forward position like the penis is now located between the thighs. There is an inward rotation of the thighs, bringing them together in the midline. And of greater significance is the change in the current excitation. Instead of flowing outward as in the case of the boy, it *turns inward* along the walls of the vagina. This is shown in the diagram as a functional invagination. Obviously this serves the function of mature sexuality and reproduction.

Embryologically, the vagina itself develops as an invagination. The word itself is taken from this process. Although the vagina is formed in early embryonic life, it doesn't become functional until the feelings or energy invades the vagina after puberty. When this happens the strong genital feelings are located deep within the vagina. These feelings can only be aroused by the full penetration of the penis. The presence of these deep feelings allows a distinction to be made between superficial and deep. This distinction is absent in the feelings of the prepubertal child. The normal development of the girl described above depends upon the undisturbed maturation of individuality and personality in the earlier stages. Neurotic factors in the family can prevent or impede the normal turning in of feeling which we described above. If, for example, the feminine role is regarded as secondary and inferior, the young girl will attempt to compensate her feeling of inadequacy by identification with boys. Thus she will become aggressively assertive rather than receptive, hard rather than soft, pushing rather than yielding. The direction of energy flow will be outward rather than inward. Instead of bypassing the clitoris to invade the vagina, genital excitation will become fixated on the surface and on the clitoris. Through this organ she can feel her identity with the male. But the vagina will remain unalive and unresponsive.

One of the difficulties which students of sex have in comprehending this process stems from a mechanical view of the sexual act. The argument is that since there are no sense corpuscles in the walls of the vagina, the latter is without feeling. On the other hand, the clitoris has many sense endings (like the penis) and it is therefore the organ of greatest phenomenon; it becomes sexual only when the excitation charges the genital organ, in this case, the vagina. Sexuality is primarily a function of movement and only secondarily a function of contact. The deeper feelings in both man and woman are mobilized by the sexual movements, voluntary and involuntary. In these movements the vagina functions like an electric coil in which the penis moves back and forth. In our vulgar language it is known as a box, a hot box, into which the energy pours. Only the relation of vagina to penis provides the setting for the orgastic discharge in both man and woman.

Let us now turn to the differences between male and female sexuality. The fact that in a man the excitation focuses upon a point which is directed outward means that he tends to be more quickly aroused genitally than the woman. This is common knowledge. It has an analogy in the property of electrical energy to focus and discharge more quickly from a point than from a flat or round surface. Second, the fact that the man has the organ of penetration gives him the initiative in instituting the sexual act. Third, since his energy is directed outward and his body is more muscularly developed, he is the aggressor in the sexual relation.

We do not mean to suggest that the woman is passive or submissive. She is as active as the man in proposing a sexual relationship. Women have their own ways of indicating their desire or willingness for sexual relations: a look, a touch, a gesture, a spoken word. In the encounter of a man with a woman it is impossible to know whose spark ignited the fire of passion. From this point on the man may become the pursuer and the woman the pursued, but the latter has her ways of keeping the chase exciting and challenging to the man. Since the woman is an individual with a well-developed personality, she is basically as aggressive as a man in life-situations. We can describe the woman's attitude as aggressively receptive. She is as eager to receive the man as he is eager to enter the woman.

However, even in this situation the desire of the man for the woman will condition her response. Thus the woman is more sexually aroused if the man is aggressive and moves forward to her. Psychologically, it is said that a woman wants to be taken, she wants to be needed, and she wants to be wanted. Therefore, she is more aroused if she senses the sexual excitation or desire in the man. Probably because of the turning inward and lack of sharp focus in her body, the woman needs the man or his image to produce a strong genital excitement. For this reason, it is understandable why primitive peoples regarded the phallus as the symbol of life and fertility. It is significant, too, that we speak of a woman's sexual arousal as a response. The woman responds to the man.

Among the animals the male assumes a dominant, covering position in the sexual act. This is true of most human relations. The dominant position (on top) means that the man sets the pace and rhythm for the sexual activity. He determines the quality of the pelvic movements in their voluntary phase, speed and strength of the thrust and withdrawal. The woman has to adapt her movements to the man's rhythm so long as he is on top. She may indicate to him by word or touch that she would like a slower or faster rhythm but it is up to him to make the changes. She cannot move counter to his movements. If she responds to his movements, his climax with its strong involuntary pelvic movements will frequently trigger her climax. The man's orgasm will generally excite the woman and bring her closer to climax. In our culture, simultaneous orgasm is rare but this is only because of neurotic disturbances which interfere with normal sexual feeling in man and woman.

On the psychological and on the social level, these differences are reflected in the woman's feeling of dependence on the man. Generally a man does not have this feeling about a woman. For in truth the woman is somewhat dependent on the man, as we have seen. One difference I didn't mention before is that his failure in sex results in her failure. The reverse is not true. Loss of the erection dooms the sexual act for both parties; loss of vaginal feeling by the woman has no such effect. Because of this dependence, a woman will react, sooner or later, consciously or unconsciously, with hostility to any weakness in a man. A woman can be sympathetic, understanding and helpful to a man in need. She will support him in every effort to overcome his difficulties or limitations. But if this doesn't work, and the weakness continues, she will either leave him or destroy him. This is the psychology of the sexes. For all the identity and equality between them, man and woman are on opposite sides of the equation. Their natural antithesis can easily degenerate into conflict or war.

It is rare to find hostility on the part of the man toward the woman for any failure in her sexual function. The man tends to take upon his shoulders the responsibility for the success of the sexual relationship. He feels that it is up to him to satisfy the woman. While I have suggested earlier that this attitude resembles the homosexual approach, we must recognize that it has some basis in the dynamics of a normal sex relationship. For the man is aware that if he were manly enough, no woman would have anything to complain of. If a woman needs at times to have her femininity affirmed by a man, it can only be done by a full-bodied man. Let me illustrate this problem with a story.

A female patient related to me her difficulties with her husband. She said: "He wanted to make love to me last night. He sidled up to me in bed then hesitantly tried to caress me. The worm! I was so disgusted, I shoved him out of the bed." I could feel her contempt for him. It angered me and I replied: "If I was your husband, I'd have beaten you up." To my surprise, she said, "I wish he had."

There is another aspect of the dependence of the woman upon the man which plays a big role in the failure of our marriages. This is the problem of romance—why does romance go out of the window in marriage?

It is a common complaint of married women that the romance has disappeared from the relationship. I have never heard this complaint from a man. Women seem to count upon men for the romantic feelings. What we seem to have in place of romance is glamour. Glamour is the feminine contribution to excitement. It is the ingredient that sparks the ads and sells the movies. But no matter how much money is spent on making a woman glamorous, it cannot sustain a relationship. It exists only as long as the woman is placed on a pedestal. But even then, the romance is missing.

Men are the bearers of romance; they are the romantic creatures. Romance, understood as the excitement of life, is an attribute of man as a fighter, hunter, adventurer, explorer, artisan, scientist or creative person. In primitive cultures (and somewhat even today), men were the dancers, the singers, the artists. They were the warriors and hunters who brought the feeling of excitement into the village while the women stayed home doing the chores and taking care of the family. In our culture there appears to be a reversal of values. Feminine values have gained the ascendancy. The home, the children and the family have become the dominant values. The whole process of earning a living is aimed at buying a home, improving it, buying furniture, raising a family, etc. These are feminine values because the home and the family are extensions of the woman. Her interests have become dominant as she herself has become idealized.

What, then, are masculine values? Adventure is a masculine value. There is less adventure in our lives and few men are engaged in adventure. Work in the sense of achievement and creation (building, for example, is a masculine activity and value). But work which is engaged in solely to earn a living becomes a chore. I believe that the loss of manhood is related somehow to this reversal of values, to the fact that men have taken on themselves the drudgery of life.

It is pretty hard for a man to be romantic if he has to catch the 7 o'clock train to New York, rush into an office, and engage in the competitive struggle to earn a buck, worry about financial security, and grab a train back at night. Entering his home tired from this activity, he is faced with jobs to be done, children to be handled, a wife to be amused. He is lucky to have an hour to himself in front of television. What romance can he offer? Even in those cases where the woman is freed from the household chores by a maid, where she has time to visit the beauty shop regularly, go to tea, play bridge or engage in civic philanthropies, she still looks to the man for romance. Romance can only exist in a situation in which the man is free to investigate the world and to bring its excitement home to his wife and family.

Now I am not advocating that the man stay at home and the woman go to work. This would be a bigger tragedy. I do suggest that a man makes a serious mistake if he loses sight of his own masculine values, if he forgets the importance of the masculine activities. An active interest in the world, in physical activities, such as sports, can do much to help a man feel that he is not simply a "drudge." But, above all, he should not be misled into the worship of the female. A man is a man in his antithesis to a woman, not in his identification with her.

Another difference between male and female sexuality is in their reactions to infidelity. A woman can tolerate sexual infidelity more easily than she can accept the withdrawal of her lover's interest in her in favor of another woman. The opposite is true of a man. A husband is more hurt by the sexual infidelity of his wife than he is by her love for another man. These are broad generalizations, of course, but they are important in the psychology of the sexes. The sexual infidelity of a wife threatens a husband in his manhood; it is felt as an insult to his pride in his ability to hold and to satisfy a woman. A cuckolded husband is an object of contempt, not pity. It is different with a woman. So long as her husband supports her in her position, she is respected by the community. Few women question their ability to satisfy a man. Their pride is based upon their ability to hold a man against the allure of another woman.

We can appreciate this difference if we realize that a man's pride is in his genital function. A man identifies with his penis as an extension of himself. The penis has an independent existence for a man in a sense as we mentioned in an earlier lecture. He refers to it as to another person, calling it Peter, John, Mon Petit Frere, him. The rejection of the penis is a more serious insult than the rejection of the person himself. Having no such appendage a woman can fixate on her breasts or *identify with her body*. A man doesn't penetrate the vagina only; he penetrates the body of the woman. The vagina is an aperture to the body. In the sense in which we spoke above, the true genital organ of a woman is not the aperture or the vagina but her body. Actually, the man doesn't penetrate the woman. Only his penis does. The penis thus becomes the symbol for that man. A woman needs no symbol for her sexual nature.

Because of this relationship to her body, a woman has a stronger sense of self, a better identification with her body than a man does. And since a woman's body is her genital organ, her sexual feelings are more intimately and directly connected with her body than the man's. She takes a greater interest in her body and spends more time on it than a man does. It is equal to a man's interest in his body and in his penis.

Seen in this light, we can say that a man has a dual aspect: his body and his penis. Does this correspond to a duality in his personality? A man belongs to the world and to the woman. His body belongs to the world; it is geared for action in the world of men. His penis belongs to the woman. With this dual relationship, a man is woman's bridge to the world. He brings the romance and excitement of the world to the woman. No woman can bring the romance of the world to a man in her nature as a woman. She can only attempt this if she has masculine attributes and engages in masculine activities.

Is there a duality in the nature of a woman, too? Nature is never one-sided. Every observation points to the fact that one thing opposes and balances another in nature. All functional relationships are complementary. They dovetail. The biology of woman is conditioned by her role as a sexual partner and as a mother; by her genital organ and by her breasts, or in the functions of sexuality and reproduction. The latter function is sometimes referred to in the third person. Thus a woman will describe her menses as "my friend has come to visit." We would not be wrong in ascribing a dual nature to the woman based on her relationship to the man and to her children. If a man is a woman's bridge to the world, she is man's bridge to the future through the children. No matter how we analyze the functions of the man and of the woman, we find that they are complementary. To gain a better idea of how these complementary functions interact, let us enlarge the tableau.

One of the poets described man as a whirlpool of dust kicked up on the face of the earth by some passing cosmic wind. In Genesis we learn that God created man by taking a piece of clay and breathing life into it. Many primitive tribes used to believe that a woman became pregnant when the spirit entered her body, from the air or from the sea. This was before the primitive learned the connection between intercourse and reproduction. Since the child came out through the vagina, it was assumed that the spirit had entered that way. In the Trobriand Islands, as reported by Malinowski, a woman who wished to become pregnant would squat in the sea, allowing the sea water to flow into her vagina, hoping that the spirit would enter her body and fertilize it.

Life on earth, as we know it, is a surface phenomenon, that is, it exists on the interface where earth and sky meet, or where water and sky meet. No life is found in the interior of the earth. We can safely assume that life is the product of the interaction of these two entities. This is true of plants who obtain minerals and fluids from the earth and solar energy from the sky. All animal life is dependent upon this process in the plant for its own energy needs. In a symbolic sense, if not actually, the basic creative process is a union of earth and sky, or elements which represent them.

Is it too much to assume in their own creative activity, sexual union, man and woman represent these two major primordial elements? In the act of sex the woman would represent the earth, while the man represents the sky. When the male covers the female or man covers a woman, it may represent the sky covering the earth. Isn't the womb a bit of earth which the woman carries within her body, waiting for the seed to be planted in it. The seed is also the spirit which comes through the air. This view is supported by two time-tested analogies. The sun is frequently thought of as impregnating the earth with its warmth, thereby bringing forth life. And the penis is often represented by a plow. Female goddesses have always been pictured as earth deities, whereas the masculine gods became established through or in connection with the worship of the sun.

The significance of this analogy for our understanding of male and female sexuality lies in the different functions which belong to each sex. The man is primarily a moving element which comes to rest in a woman. The woman is the more stationary element who is there to receive the man. We have said that a man belongs to the world and to the woman. But he can be in neither if he isn't in both. If a man isn't in the world or part of it, he cannot belong to the woman, nor properly relate to her. But if he cannot function as a man to a woman, he is not really a man in the world of men. Women have this dual relationship to life, too. She can only function as a woman to a man if she also functions as his home and as the mother of his children.

Let me say immediately that I am not proclaiming that woman's place is in the home. Kirche, kuche and kinder is Nazi ideology, which places a woman in an inferior position, thereby destroying the natural harmony of the sexual relationship. The same fallacy occurs when the woman's role as a homemaker becomes the dominant activity. A woman doesn't *make* a home, a woman *is* the home. The home grows out of the woman's personality. She cannot make it. If she does not feel in herself that she is the home, that it is to her a man returns and that it is out of her that children grow, she has lost the sense of herself as a woman. A woman creates a home by her warmth and presence; that is, by accepting herself as a woman.

We have said earlier that a man should not lose his identification with masculine values if he wishes to be a man. But the same holds true for the woman. Envy of the man and the attempt to capture the masculine role will only result for a woman in the loss of her true self— her feminine nature. Each must have pride in his own nature and each must have respect for the nature of the other. Respect is the other side of pride. A person who doesn't respect another can have no pride in himself. The man who can earn the respect of the woman for his activity in the world will gain her sexual feelings. The woman who is respected as the spirit which informs the home and the children will also be the object of the man's desire and passion.

A healthy sexual relationship is founded on mutual respect for the differences between a man and a woman. A successful marriage is based upon mutual respect for their complementary roles in life. We said earlier in this lecture that the one quality which guarantees a good upbringing for children is respect: first, respect for the individuality of the young child; second, respect for the personality of the growing child; and, third, respect for the sexuality of the youth. Respect creates pride which in its natural form is self-esteem. Without pride in one's self and one's sexuality, one would not have the ego strength to sustain the excitation until it explodes in orgasm and ecstasy.

One word more. The biological function of the woman as home and mother is best represented by the specific act of breast feeding. The degree to which women in our culture have abandoned this basic mammalian function, the one function which is distinctive of the animal order to which they belong, is paralleled by the degree to which they have given up their womanhood and lost their sexuality. If there is one function which furthers the development of individuality in the infant, it is nursing. Nothing interferes with genitality so much as the persistence of unfulfilled oral longing. If our men are inadequate as men it is fundamentally because they have not been fulfilled as babies. And if it is true that the trouble with women is men, it is also true that the trouble with men was women.

7

The Will to Live and the Wish to Die

We have said many times that character structure is a survival
mechanism. This means that a person's particular neurotic character
is developed in childhood as a means of surviving. Whether or not it
is actually true that the person would not have survived if he had not
developed his neurotic character, we cannot know. We do know that the
resistance to giving up on character, though unconscious, is enormous.
The person behaves as if stepping out of character is a step into the
uncertainty of life or death. We understand that no one would accept
the limitations of neurosis unless he believed it was the only way to
safeguard his life or his sanity.

But the threats to the integrity of the individual which led to the
formation of the neurotic character structure occurred in childhood. Why,
then, is that structure maintained with such tenacity in adult life? The
patient himself recognizes that the threats are no longer present. What
forces are operative in his personality to keep him neurotic, to maintain
the character structure, to resist the natural tendency of the body and
mind to heal itself? Given the magnitude of this resistance, these must
be very powerful forces.

Every experienced therapist knows that resistance occurs on many
levels of the neurotic personality, from the most superficial to the most
profound. We are all familiar with the fact that every neurotic derives

certain secondary gains from his illness which he is reluctant to give up. We know that there is a basic resentment in neurotics stemming from the fact that they have always been made to feel wrong. A neurotic could very well say to his therapist, "Why am I always the one who has to change? Why am I always the one who is wrong?" But there are also some very deep resistances, one of which I would like to explore in this paper. That one is the will to live.

It may seem strange to regard the will to live as a resistance to therapy. Certainly the will to die is a resistance. It is almost impossible to do any effective therapy with a patient who is intent on committing suicide. The customary practice in such cases is to confine the person in a controlled environment until the impulse or intent to kill himself subsides. It would also be helpful to get the person to see that this impulse is really the result of turning his anger or rage against himself. If it can be turned outward again, the impulse to self-destruction is reduced. But how can the will to live be regarded as a resistance to therapy?

The answer depends upon an understanding of the expression "Will to live." The will is an instrument of the ego since it represents the ego's ability to control the motility of the body; that is, to control the action of the voluntary muscles. Every act of will is a statement of determination. For example, the statement, "I will do it," could also be rendered as "I am determined to do it." Both statements imply an obstacle against which the will is operative. Where there is no obstacle to an impulse, the will is unnecessary. I do not need my will to do something I want to do. It requires no will power to eat when one is hungry or to sleep when one is sleepy. It is rather that one needs to use the will if one wishes to resist the impulse to eat when one is hungry or to sleep when one is sleepy. Doing what comes naturally requires no conscious effort or will. Isn't living something that comes naturally to all living things? Why, then, does one need to use one's will or to be determined—to live? One doesn't unless there is a wish to die. In that case, survival might require the use of the will.

I first became aware of this problem when a patient remarked, "If I breathe, I will die." I had the feeling that she was expressing a deep self-perception. But how is that possible? What sense does it make? Breathing makes a person more alive. How can it lead to death?

The answer to this question is very important to an understanding of resistance. The more alive a person is, the more he will feel. And if the feelings he has are a deep despair, which is intolerable, or an intense pain which is unbearable, he will do everything possible to avoid making contact with them; namely, not breathe deeply so as not to feel much. In the case above, the person had come close to dying as a baby. She related the story as follows: "I was an only child. It seems that because of that, my mother was determined not to spoil me. When I was about two months old, my mother and grandmother decided that they would no longer rock me to sleep. It was an indulgence that would spoil me. So they put me in my crib in a room and closed the door. I cried but my mother was not going to give in to me. She would let me cry myself out. I cried for hours—my grandmother was going crazy, but my mother refused to let her go into my room, Finally, I stopped crying and my mother said, 'See.' They opened the door and saw. I was blue. I had vomited and was choking on the vomitus."

The amazing thing about this story is that my patient heard it from her mother who told it with pride. She had not given in to the child. It was not the mother who learned a lesson from this incident, but the child. If you want to live, don't want too much, don't feel too much, don't breathe too much.

Generally children don't die if they are left to "cry it out." But the point at which they finally stop crying and fall asleep is a state of complete exhaustion. At this point the child is close to death in the feeling that he has reached the limit of his energy. Fortunately, sleep supervenes, not death. But the lesson is not always learned immediately. The child may cry himself to sleep on successive nights, each time reaching the stage of exhaustion more quickly. Finally, he will go to sleep alone without crying, but he has experienced a closeness to death which he cannot forget. And in the interest of survival, he will suppress his longing for contact and love, so as not to cry for something he cannot get.

The next insight into this problem came as the result of an observation during a breathing exercise. In that exercise, the patient lies on the stool and breathes out as deeply as possible. At the end of the expiration, the patient holds against breathing in. To do this, he has to use his will since the normal tendency would be to breathe in after a short pause. The length of the holding against breathing provides some evidence of the patient's structure. If the patient breathes in immediately after the completion of the expiration, it denotes a panic about letting down and an insecurity about letting go. Many persons experience the panic which they explain as: "I need air," or "I feel that if I don't breathe in, I'll die." Of course, one doesn't die so quickly from not breathing. The body has a two-to-three-minute reserve of air. Besides, when the need for air is acute, the body will take over and breathe against any conscious effort to inhibit it. If pushed to the extreme, the person will faint and start breathing again.

We know that the breath can be held for fairly long periods. I believe ten minutes is the record. Anyone who has practiced underwater swimming knows that the breath can be held. But that is not the same as our exercise. Underwater swimmers hold the air in after a deep inspiration. In the above exercise, the air is held out after a deep expiration.

In doing this exercise, some people hold the air out for what seems like an inordinate length of time. On a couple of occasions, I became nervous. One person passed out, slid off the stool and went into a convulsive reaction. It lasted only a few seconds. His breathing became very full and he later said that he felt great. Many people fall into a middle group between these two extremes.

When people hold the breath out a very long time, one has the impression that the body's desire to live is weak. The insight I had was that on some level of the personality, the individual has a wish to die. When the will to live is immobilized by the exercise, the desire to die becomes evident. In almost all cases my impression is confirmed by the patient. Now the reason for the inability of the first group to hold the air out becomes clear. They, too, have a wish to die which frightens them very much. It is countered by a strong will to live, whereas in the second group, the will to live is weak. A strong will to live implies a strong wish to die, else why such a strong will? It also becomes clear why a strong will to live is a resistance. The person is afraid to let go of his will because it counters a wish to die.

There are, as I said, some people in a middle group whose will is not strongly manifested because there is no big wish to die. This group can hold the air out for a time long enough to excite a powerful gasp for air. This gasp represents the wish to live expressed in the intensity with which air is sucked into the body. The throat opens wide to take in as much air as possible. Following this gasp, the patient's breathing is very deep and full and very often it is followed by deep sobs. The crying is a sense of release from the *fear of death* associated with the *wish to die*.

On the deepest level of the personality in all organisms there is a desire to live which is an expression of the positive life force in an individual. The desire to live is the biological phenomenon which motivates the instinct for self-preservation. It is the core of one's being. It is manifested in all the life-maintaining functions of the body: the beating of the heart, the peristaltic waves of the intestines, the expansion and contraction of respiration plus all the myriad activities of the different organs, tissues and cells. Breathing is the most visible of these functions and can serve, therefore, as an indication of the strength of this life force. How strongly a person breathes in reflects the strength of his desire to live. Since breathing in is a process of sucking air, what we measure is the intensity of the sucking impulse. Any childhood experiences which weaken this impulse reduce the strength of the desire to live. Any exercise, such as the above, which mobilizes and strengthens this impulse, increases a person's energy and desire to live.

Therapy aims to help a person make direct contact with this life force so that it is available for personal fulfillment. But to make this contact, the patient has to get through the two more superficial layers of his personality; namely, the will to live and the wish to die. The following diagram shows the layering. But we must recognize that the will to live derives its energy from the life force and the wish to live. And since the will to live offers survival but not fulfillment, it weakens the underlying wish to live.

Persons in whom the will to live is strong can be called survivors. They are characterized either by significant rigidities or a set, determined, often-grim jaw, or both. They can survive but they cannot find fulfillment since their energy is totally committed to survival. In effect, they remain at the level of pain and despair which characterized the original trauma and led to the wish to die. In other words, the wish to die is constantly reinforced by the lack of personal fulfillment (love) due to the preoccupation with survival. This means that a patient must surrender his will to live so he can experience his wish to die, go through it, and contact his life force at its very core: the impulse to breathe.

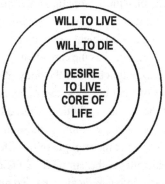

Fig. 1

A good example of this process can be seen in the following report of a therapeutic session at a workshop. I was struck by an expression of death on the face of a young man as he was lying over the stool.

He was simply doing some breathing exercises. As I passed by, I remarked, "You have a look of death on your face."

He came up to work with me later. Standing before the group he commented on my observation and said, "I have been preoccupied with death lately. My wife committed suicide about three months ago." But the expression on his face told a different story—of an encounter with death much earlier in life. His set jaw betrayed a strong will to live.

I suggested that he try the exercise described above of holding the air out. It generally takes several attempts before a patient can muster the courage to stay without breathing long enough to mobilize a significant gasp. That was the case with this patient. When his throat opened and the gasp broke through, he began to sob deeply saying, "I want to live, I want to live."

After the exercise, I asked him if he had come close to death. "Yes," he said. "I almost died when I was a baby. In fact, the doctors didn't expect me to live. I wouldn't eat and kept losing weight."

I asked him what had happened at that time in his life. He said, "My mother weaned me."

The patient's set jaw expressed two aspects of the same attitude of determination: One, that he wasn't going to reach out for his mother with his mouth; the frustration he had experienced as a child had been too painful. And two, that he was determined to survive, which he would accomplish by not reaching out to a woman, thereby avoiding the pain of rejection. But living on a survival level, he was not far removed from death and it showed on his face.

I suggested that he try to discharge the pain of the past and present which fed into his wish to die. He could do this by reaching out for his mother. He lay on the mattress and extended his arms and his lips, calling to his mother at the same time. I applied a steady pressure to the tight muscles of his jaw. He broke into such heartrending sobs that all of us present could sense the agony of the man (and the baby) at the loss of his world, the breast of his mother, which represented joy and fulfillment to him. When it was over, he said that he felt so much better, so much freer than before. He had known the story of his illness but he had never connected it with the loss of the breast. The deep crying had also washed the look of death and pain from his face.

253

Not every case is as dramatic as this one. In many cases, it is not easy for the patient to get past the will to live and experience the wish to die. The fear of death is too strong to permit this confrontation. One has to work with a patient for a long time helping him to gain the courage to go through the valley of death to reach the sunshine on the other side. I assure my patients that they will not die in this confrontation. They survived the real experience when they were younger and more helpless. With time and encouragement, I can get most of them to try the exercise. When it works, its effect is positive and powerful.

There are probably other ways to approach the problem of the wish to die which must be similar to what Freud described as the death instinct. The important thing is not the technique one uses, but the understanding of the problem.

How common is the wish to die? In a culture such as ours where survival is a major preoccupation of people, one can suspect that it is quite common.

Here are some examples from my practice.

This is a patient I have worked with for many years. Her complaint was a lack of feeling. She felt numb. From an emotional point of view, her body was dead. Intensive body work in the therapy sessions, the exercise classes, and at home, slowly brought her body back to life. Her will to survive and even to get well was strong, but she was aware, as was I, of an underlying wish to die. She expressed it as follows: "I'm afraid I'm just going to die. I'd put the brake on my heart and that would be it."

I had her do the exercise of holding against breathing in. She had tried it before with no success. This time, she was able to hold the air out for a little longer, although she gave no gasp when she breathed in. However, she had a very strong sensation of being unable to breathe. She cried out, "I can't breathe. I'm choking, I can't breathe." I could see that she had difficulty breathing. Her chest and throat looked so tight I could understand her difficulty.

When I commented on my observation, she said, "I've felt this tightness in my throat and chest for years. I sensed that I couldn't breathe. I couldn't get a simple, deep breath because there was such pain in my diaphragm. I don't know how I survived. But I know I died a long time ago."

The death that occurred is the emotional death, the numbness, the cutting off of feeling. This is done because of the intolerable pain. Such pain leads to a wish to die. Cutting off feeling is a compromise between the wish to die and the will to live.

Another patient, Roger, who is also a survivor, said, "There is such a sense of frustration and helplessness that I feel I could almost roll over and die. Well, not exactly. Death is too violent, too final, too destructive. I would like to turn off living for a while so I could get a break.

"Seven or eight years ago, I was so depressed, I had no appetite, no desire. I don't feel depressed now, but I feel, Jesus, I'm just wasting time."

Roger has a body that is extremely rigid, and without feeling. Despite his hopelessness and frustration, he cannot cry. He cannot break down, figuratively, in terms of crying and literally, in terms of his rigidity. To break down is to give in to a despair that is nigh unto death.

Jane is another patient whom I regard as a survivor. She has a strong and extremely tense jaw. There has been a lot of pain in her life with relatively little pleasure. Her statement is, "I don't want to live if I have to live the way I do." Yet she holds on as if for dear life, as if letting go would mean her death. When she did let go in some therapy sessions, it evoked an intense pain in the lower right-hand quadrant of her abdomen. I associate that pain with a holding against her despair and her sexuality. Her sexuality is connected with a sense of betrayal by her father which was so painful that it took a very strong effort of will to continue living.

Many years ago, I treated a man whose stated attitude was, "You can live as long as you want to." I thought he was kidding himself since he didn't seem such a healthy person. He suffered from arthritis which had actually crippled him. Also, he was a rather heavy smoker, despite his recognition that each cigarette was a coffin nail. One of the problems of this patient was some degree of sexual impotence. Although very successful in his business, he was in effect, a castrated man. In his youth, he was dominated by an overbearing father of whom he was very much afraid.

I did not make much progress with this patient. One day I told him that he would have to confront his father—in his feelings, since his father was no longer living. He never could muster any anger against his father. My statement seemed to shock him.

I never saw this patient again. He missed the next two appointments and I had a suspicion that something was wrong. When I called his home I learned that the weekend after his last visit he had discovered a swelling in his neck. He went to a doctor who ordered a biopsy which showed that it was malignant. He died within three months. Now I understand the meaning of his remark. When a person dies, it denotes the wish to die on a biological level. It can be said, therefore, that the person lived as long as he wished. But why did it happen then? What undermined his will to live? The answer has to be that his energy system collapsed to a point where the life force was insufficient to sustain basic life functions. This collapse is characteristic of cancer, the predisposition to which is emotional resignation. (See the chapter, "Stress and Illness" for a more complete statement of this concept.) I would guess that my patient gave up at the thought of facing what must have seemed to him an impossible challenge. (Some time later, a cancer patient with whom I was working, expressed the thought, "If I fight my mother, I will die. If I don't fight her, I will die." Her doom seemed unavoidable, and she did die.)

If I would work with this patient today, I would be more conscious of his wish to die since it was expressed implicitly in the statement, "You can live as long as you want to," and in other aspects of his personality. Then instead of having him confront his father, I would have him confront his wish to die. I believe that this is the only way to deal with such problems. I don't think that it's possible to help a cancer patient overcome his illness unless he can first accept that the illness expresses his wish to die. In that way, instead of trying to overcome his despair, the patient can work into it and through it.

It has been found statistically that cancer often develops in an older person following the loss of a loved person. It is assumed, and rightly so, that the stress of the loss produces the illness. Many researchers recognize the fact that this loss in later life repeats a similar trauma that happened in childhood; namely, the loss of the mother or her love expressed in the loss of the breast or of physical contact with the mother's body. This later loss activates the wish to die, which had been suppressed by the will to live.

This awareness has led me to the realization that many serious illnesses are related to an unconscious wish to die. The relationship is not a direct one, however. People do not make themselves sick because they wish to die. As we saw, people have an even stronger desire to live, to experience the joy of life. Unfortunately, that desire is weakened by the will to live which puts the individual under stress and maintains him in a state of pain and despair. If the person comes under additional stress or experiences a new pain of an emotional nature, his resistance weakens and illness develops. I have seen this happen to a young woman following the break-up of a love affair. In the course of her illness, she was quite conscious of the wish to die. However, she did not connect this wish to an earlier life experience which would have placed her present situation in perspective. In consequence, her recovery was unduly delayed.

The individual in whom the will to live is strong, is in a state of struggle. His will is fighting against his wish to die. That struggle must and does deplete his energy eventually undermining his will. Many persons are in a state of exhaustion as a result. I'll never forget the man who, while lying over the stool breathing, suddenly burst into tears with the exclamation, "I am so tired I could die." He admitted his fatigue, but I've seen many patients who denied their exhaustion, who set their jaws and struggled on, who felt that to stop was to die. I have another patient who has been in a state of exhaustion for a long time, but unable to give in to it and cry. It took years of work to bring him to the realization of the struggle he was engaged in. But finally, he did come to that realization.

He said, "Life is such a struggle. If I give up the struggle, I give up life."

"I don't know how to live for me. I am involved in raising my family, getting my children married, working, etc. All my life has been a continual effort to justify my existence because I wasn't supposed to be there. My mother didn't want another child but if there was to be one, she wanted a girl. When I was born, she said, 'Take him away. He's not mine.'"

Why his mother told him that story, I don't know. It placed such a burden upon him.

On another occasion, he said, "If I stop struggling, I couldn't survive. I have to earn my way. I have to be a good boy and do what they want or I'll be abandoned. Without my struggling, everything would collapse."

How long can he go on struggling before his health breaks down? He is already in a state of exhaustion and doesn't really feel in good health. Yet medical exams reveal nothing wrong since the doctors do not see his state of exhaustion. I am worried for him.

I am convinced that many illnesses happen to people because they cannot accept their exhaustion and so continue to struggle. Many of you are familiar with the story of Norman Cousins' illness which he reported in a book entitled *The Anatomy of an Illness*. It came on suddenly, and was nearly fatal. He cured himself by the unusual regime of laughter and an extremely high dosage of Vitamin C. His account of the events just prior to the onset of the illness reveals the stress he was under, the extreme fatigue he sensed. This extreme exhaustion is rarely due to present conditions. Soldiers in battle may become so tired, they can't move. But such tiredness rarely results in illness. Their unconscious wish to die may be expressed by careless exposure to the enemy. The exhaustion that produces illness is a chronic condition stemming from a strong will to live which, to insure survival, is unconsciously active in the suppression of feeling.

I have written that all patients go through a phase of exhaustion on their way to recovery. In reality, they become conscious of their exhaustion as they give up the neurotic struggle. The exhaustion also helps the recovery. Feeling exhausted, they cannot continue the neurotic struggle. They feel the need to recover their spirits, renew their energy; in other words, to convalesce. This points the way to the handling of the resistance represented by the will to live.

Treatment

In view of the foregoing, it is to be expected that every patient will present some resistance to the therapeutic process in the interest of survival. Our role as therapists is to understand this resistance, its nature, its origin and its present-day function. Understanding is the key to the therapeutic process. The patient's role is to gain this understanding and with our help, to confront his wish to die. Through that confrontation, he can touch the life force connected to the wish to live. The breathing exercise described above is a good technique for this confrontation. I had occasion to test this out recently with a patient with whom I have worked for several years with very positive results.

One of this patient's problems was a feeling that he could not have what he wanted. It was not a conscious feeling, but one manifested in his behavior. The feeling was focused primarily upon a woman. As we examined the feeling, it turned out that he was not allowed to need a woman. Of course, this feeling stemmed from his experience with his mother. In the interest of survival he denied his need, and if he found some woman who was prepared to love him, he had to reject her. This issue was touched peripherally in the years of therapy, but never confronted because other, more pressing, conflicts in his life demanded attention. As these other conflicts were resolved, he began to feel good, but it did not hold up. He still felt tormented by a need that he could not accept.

The torment, or torture, of this patient, was physically as well as psychologically determined. His pelvis was too tight, his chest too bound, and his throat too constricted. For all the physical work we had done (and he worked with the stool at home, too), these tensions had not been significantly reduced. I asked him to do the exercise of holding his breath out. He was able to hold against breathing for a good time, but his inspiration was weak. A second try was a little better, but not strong enough. He was lying over the stool breathing. I suggested that he say, "I want to live." To my surprise and his, he had difficulty saying these words. As he said, "I can't say it," he began to cry. With the crying, his throat opened and his breathing became deeper and stronger. The crying was an expression of his wish to live. But crying was not easy for him, either. Having been denied the right to need, he lost the right to cry. His need now was to cry so deeply that his breath would come in gasps.

There is only one treatment for the conflict between the wish to die and the will to live, and that is deep sobbing. By deep sobbing, I mean a full-throated belly crying. When a person cries in that way, one can observe that each sob is a pulse of life that flows through the body and into the pelvis. Such crying releases the pain that underlies the wish to die. That pain is in the tight jaw, the constricted throat, the held chest and the sucked-in belly. These tensions block the expression of the longing for love and for life. In the interest of survival, they close the person off. But in doing so, they structure the pain into the body. As long as he is closed off, the person doesn't feel the pain. All he feels is a deep sense of frustration and hopelessness which maintains the unconscious wish to die. But to open, to reach out and to express one's wanting with all one's desire makes the pain come alive. There is no pain in death which is the great appeal of death for so many people. There is no pain in life if one is fully alive, for then the flow of energy and feeling is free and unrestricted. The pain is in coming alive, in the flow of energy and feeling into tight or dead areas of the body in the effort to break out of one's chains. In the final analysis, it is the fear of this pain which leads to resistance in therapy.

The pain is associated with the wish to die as the following report indicates. This is a 32-year-old secretary named Mary, in whom the manifestation of oral deprivation is quite marked. Her head and face appear undercharged. The head is small in relation to the body, the face looks weak. Her sternum is collapsed and her diaphragm extremely tense, making it difficult for her to take a deep breath. Her respiratory weakness is reflected in a thin voice. Her legs are normal in shape, but not strong.

In her first session, she related a recurrent dream. "I am lying on my side and a man is making an incision into my back with a razor blade. Sometimes he is my doctor, sometimes he is my guru. The pain is always excruciating. I want to scream but I can't get any sound out. I feel helpless, then I wake up."

Mary's interpretation was "I want someone to cut me open and take the pain away." She had been involved with therapists and gurus for many years in a desperate effort to get the pain out of her. It was still there. I was another desperate attempt to get away from it. Unfortunately, there is only one way to get free from her pain and that is through death. The procedure of cutting her open to release her from the pain is in itself excruciatingly painful. This is not to say that her situation is hopeless. There is one thing she can do which could lead to a resolution of the conflict underlying the pain, and that is to understand that the pain is a product of conflict and what the conflict is about. But to do that, she must accept her pain and see it as a manifestation of the life force in her. Many efforts to get rid of the pain always involved procedures that diminished her life force. But this could only be a temporary measure because when her longing reasserted itself, the pain returned.

Mary was aware of the connection between her pain and her longing. At the time she consulted me, both her pain and her longing were focused upon a man who was withdrawing from his relationship with her. She was aware that if she could withdraw from him and cut off her feelings, the pain would go away. But this she could not do. His withdrawal was so threatening that she said, "I'd rather have the pain than be abandoned." The fear of abandonment was terrifying. It could only be because in her mind it was associated with death. She had come close to death as an infant. "When I was born, my mother almost died. They said her milk turned to poison. I became almost like a skeleton. Then when I was nine months old, I had food poisoning."

The basic conflict in Mary's personality is between the desire to live with its accompanying pain and the wish to die. Since her wish to die is strong, her will to live is equally strong. The latter is expressed in a very tight jaw. While this tight jaw represents her will to live, it also locks into her body the pain of living and loving. She cannot scream because it is too painful and she cannot breathe deeply for the same reason. It is necessary, in my opinion, to work with this tight jaw to open her breathing and release her screaming. That means pressure has to be applied to the tight jaw muscles so that they will let go. This is always a painful procedure, but if the patient is encouraged to focus upon breathing, the pain is tolerable because the muscles do let go. I also encourage patients to try to scream which they can do sometimes. The screaming also reduces the pain.

Screaming is essential to health. It is the strongest expression of the desire to live. Healthy babies will scream whenever their desires are frustrated and as long as they can scream, the frustration does not become locked into the body. Screaming expresses pain and, therefore, releases pain. It has been used in Bioenergetic Analysis long before it was discovered to be an effective therapeutic tool by Arthur Janov. Let me say that it is not as easy to get men to scream as women, but they are by nature equally capable of screaming.

To work with screaming bioenergetically, one has to understand the muscular and energetic dynamics. The scream is produced by a sudden expulsion of air. That happens when the throat, which is holding against the expiration, lets go and opens wide. The muscles involved are the anterior scalenes, the stylohyoid, and the digastricus. Actually, all the muscles of the area play some part in the various functions of the mouth and throat; screaming, crying, breathing, sucking. The gasp is the reverse side of the scream in that it is produced by a sudden opening of the throat at the beginning of inspiration of air. And both screaming and gasping are related to the function of sucking. Thus, by releasing the scream, one can open up the sudden sucking in of air which we describe as a gasp and which I call an expression of the desire to live.

In many cases, I can produce a scream by applying pressure to the anterior scalene muscles while the patient is making a sound. The pressure produces a sudden release of the holding which allows the scream to break through. If one can get the patient to utter several long sustained screams, it will generally lead to deep sobbing with strong sucking actions in the throat. As long as the screaming is in progress, the patient feels no pain from the pressure. Often, the screaming will continue long after I have removed my pressure. I believe the critical area where the sucking is blocked is at the back of the mouth where it joins the throat.

The screaming and sobbing release the pain of the suppressed longing, because it allows the free flow of the impulse to want and to reach out. Frustration is due to an inability to fully express one's impulses and not to the lack of response to them. When I got Mary to scream, using this technique, she always felt stronger. She also reported some pain in her head as the energy of the scream charged that part. But this pain subsided quickly. Once a patient can get the screaming opened up, he or she can begin to fight for their rights. The patient can kick the bed screaming "Why" or "No" or "Leave me alone." It can then move into more aggressive expressions such as "Give it to me," and "I want it." This was something Mary could not do. She had no sense that she could make any demands for herself. She wanted to love and be loved but since she could not demand it, she hoped to get love by "being there" for the other person which, in effect, is a surrender of the self. But no one can really love a person who has denied his self and so she always reproduced her primal pain. Mary could be there for others, but never for herself. This is not an uncommon problem.

It became clear to me that the interpretation of Mary's dream was incomplete. If we are talking about the pain associated with suppressed longing, it would be experienced along the front of the body. That pain would not be diminished by an incision in the back. The pain in the back is related to blocked anger. That is an emotion which Mary does not allow herself to experience because it could lead to a loss of contact with the love object. Her role, as she sees it, is to be understanding and she tries to be understanding even when she is abused as she was in the relationship immediately past.

Yet Mary is angry. That is the normal response to abuse and Mary was abused as a child by her father and as a woman by men. But she regards her anger as a threat to her life situation, rather than as a support for it. Her aim has been to diminish her anger, hoping that this would eliminate the pain. The incision in her back had this function. The gurus she has consulted and the Sufi practices she followed have had as their aim to reduce her anger and, temporarily, they succeeded. But as long as her longing for love is frustrated, she will be in pain. Necessarily, the pain will evoke anger, and she will be in the same situation as before. It seems that the conflict between the will to live and the wish to die cannot be satisfactorily resolved unless the person's anger is mobilized.

In the earlier part of this paper, I emphasized the importance of opening the throat through breathing, screaming and crying to allow the wish to live full expression. As we saw, that expression was manifested in the gasp in the sucking in of air. We have to ask—what sustains the wish to live? It was weakened in infancy and childhood by the lack of parental response to the need for love and nurturing. The pain of that deprivation gave rise to a wish to die, which was then countered by a will to live. The process of therapy is to go backwards, reversing the process that led to the development of the neurotic character. Theoretically, that would lead the person back to the state of dependency and to the infantile need for nurturing and support. Of course, this need can no longer be fulfilled. I say "of course" but it may not be so evident to others. An infant is fulfilled on the oral level, an adult only on the genital level. Sucking on a teat is a nurturing act for a child, but a sexual act for a man.

The differences between the child and the adult must be recognized if we are to help people find some fulfillment in life. Thus a child feels lovable when he is loved, but an adult feels lovable when he is able to love. Fulfillment as an adult represents the ability to function fully on the adult level. In effect, fulfillment is the realization of one's potential for being. Frustration results when one is blocked or inhibited from being fully who one is; that is, from fully expressing one's feelings or fully functioning on all levels of the personality. It follows, therefore, that denying one's anger or restraining one's aggression limits the possibility of fulfillment and produces frustration.

Loving, as I pointed out in *The Language of the Body,* is an aggressive act. It is not just wanting or reaching out, it is also taking in. To love someone is to take them into one's heart. One does have to be open so the other person can enter, but being open is not enough. Loving is not a passive process. The aggressive component of this function is located largely in the muscles of the back of the body; the same muscles that are involved in anger. Denying one's anger leads to a reduction in the aggression necessary to fulfill the function of love. And just as aggression is a component of love, so loving is an aspect of aggression including anger. We get angry only at those persons towards whom we have some positive feelings. If we are indifferent or negative towards a person, we tend to avoid them. In anger, we move towards them. I often point out to patients that our tender feelings are represented by the left arm and hand; our aggressive feelings, including anger, by our right arm. Cutting off our right arm by denying our anger would not produce any fulfillment.

Why would a person deny the validity of anger? If a child is taught that his anger would lead to his rejection, he will necessarily attempt to suppress that reaction. Since children need to be loved, they will make certain sacrifices to insure that love. We know that parents discourage or will not tolerate any expression of anger by their children, especially if it is directed toward them. But I wonder if there isn't another possible explanation. If a child undergoes a severe deprivation of love and nurturing in infancy, how much anger can he feel or muster? In that early state of helplessness, isn't crying the only response he can make? He can also scream. I recall an incident from the life of my son. When he was about five months of age, my wife and I left him with a friend to do an urgent errand. We left only after all his needs were taken care of and he seemed content. However, we had only gone several minutes and were about two blocks away from the apartment we were living in when we heard a loud scream. We both knew immediately that it was Fred and we returned home. He had a powerful scream. But if a child is left to scream without response, his screaming will become weaker. His wish to live will slowly turn into a wish to die. He might mobilize the will to live. That is all his rudimentary ego can do. To feel angry and either to express it or contain it is beyond the capability of an infant. It requires a higher degree of muscular coordination than is available.

I believe it is necessary for all patients to be able to feel and express anger for both the abuse and the deprivation they suffered. I shall not describe the various techniques I use to help patients reach this objective. With Mary, I had some help from life. She came in one day and reported that she had been mugged. She fought back without thinking. But even as we discussed the events and her reaction, she did not feel any anger toward her assailants. She tried to explain their behavior to justify their actions. However, I could help her mobilize some anger towards me, slight though it was. And I made her realize how she had castrated herself, in a sense. Experiencing some anger made her feel so much better. It reduced her pain.

The problems of all patients are complicated. There is no simple answer to their difficulties. But we are not looking for answers. We are seeking to understand. I have come to understand that the will to survive may prolong life, but it cannot fulfill life. Fulfillment may require that one take some risks. The will to live can be an obstacle to risk-taking or growth. But if a person gives up the will to live, what protection does he have? How can he insure his survival to whatever degree such insurance is possible? My answer to that question is: by becoming a fighter. A fighter risks his life and may lose it, but I have seen survivors lose theirs, too. A fighter, however, has a chance to fulfill his potential for being.

A fighter is not a person looking for trouble. He is an individual who knows that he has a right to be, a right to love and a right to fulfillment. He will fight if anyone denies his rights. In Bioenergetic terms, a fighter may be defined as a person who has his aggression available—to support and realize his wish to live and love.

The Voice of the Body

8

Horror: The Face of Unreality
and
Self-Expression vs. Survival

LECTURE I. HORROR: THE FACE OF UNREALITY

Introduction

The subject of horror first arose several years ago in connection with a patient that Miki Kronold and I were treating. He was a highly educated young man, an assistant professor at one of the colleges; his primary complaint was depression. Physically he had a well-shaped body, a little shorter than average height, with few signs of any major personality disorder except that in some way his head didn't seem to go with his body. There was nothing unusual about his head, he had fairly regular features, but I sensed that head and body weren't connected.

We had considerable difficulty with this patient in that we were unable to evoke any emotional response from him. The sounds he made reminded me strongly of old Jews at the wailing wall but when I pointed this out to him, it caused no feeling or association. To remove the mask-like quality of his face, pressure was applied on the cheeks alongside his nose, while he opened his eyes wide. This brought out a strong expression of fear, but he didn't feel fear. In response to all my maneuvers he constantly remarked, "I don't feel anything."

He described his childhood situation as follows: He was the youngest child in a family of three children, the older two being girls. As far back as he remembers his mother and father did not get along well together. The mother screamed at his father, often becoming quite hysterical. His father would fly into a violent rage, occasionally breaking things and sometimes beating one of the girls. My patient saw this happen but felt powerless to intervene. He did not recall his father's hitting him. When he discussed his background my patient spoke logically and clearly but without any emotional reaction to the events he described.

We could account for his lack of feeling by assuming that he had cut off his perception of what went on in his body. He did this by dissociating what went on in his head, namely, the function of perception, from his bodily experience. This was related to the seeming lack of connection between his body and his head. No matter how much his body got charged up through breathing and movement, it didn't affect his head. Discussing this case, Miki and I came to the conclusion that such a situation could only be produced by an experience of horror.

Horror is a new term in bioenergetics. It does not appear in the spectrum of emotions which I presented in my book, *Pleasure*. On the other hand, terror, which is often used as a synonym for horror, occurs often in my writings as the extremity of fear. If one reads *The Betrayal of the Body*, it will be seen that the schizoid personality develops as a reaction to terror, not horror. What is the difference between the two?

The dictionary gives us some help. It says that terror implies an intense fear which is somewhat prolonged and may refer to imagined or future dangers. Horror implies a sense of shock at a danger which is also evil and the danger may be to others rather than to oneself. There are two major distinctions. Terror is related to fear, which is an emotional reaction; horror lacks this connection. Second, in terror, the danger is directed at the self; in horror, the danger is directed at others.

These differences can be illustrated with a few simple examples. If we witness an automobile accident in which one or more persons are badly injured, we would describe the experience as horrible. However, if one is involved in such an accident, the immediate sensation before the crash would be one of terror. One is horrified by a brutal attack on others but terrified if the attack is directed at oneself. Thus combatants in a war would speak of its terrors while non-combatants would speak of its horrors.

If terror is an intense fear, horror has no such component. The witness to a horror is not necessarily frightened. He may also be frightened fearing some personal attack in which case he would also experience a degree of terror but this is an added element. The essence of horror is the "sense of shock," although I don't think that is quite the right term. Terror ends in a real state of shock. The organism is paralyzed with terror as if frozen. The body becomes numb to spare the organism the pain of the attack. This happens when a predator attacks and kills its prey. The mind, however, remains alert until unconsciousness occurs. In a state of horror the body is relatively unaffected since the attack is not directed at the self. The effect of horror is primarily upon the mind, which is not shocked but stunned.

Horror stuns the mind. It paralyzes the mental functions as terror paralyzes the physical ones. One can walk away from a scene of horror seemingly unaffected physically but incapable of thinking about anything but the horror and really just going over it again and again.

This raises another question. Why does horror stun the mind? What is it about horror that has this effect? I think the essential element is that a horror is unbelievable. Not every unbelievable occurrence is a horror but every horror is unbelievable. The mind cannot comprehend the logic or meaning of the event. It doesn't make sense. It shouldn't be happening.

I shall offer another example of horror to illustrate this aspect. A mother walking with her six-year-old son was mugged and brutally beaten in New York. The little boy looked on in horror. He wasn't hurt. In his mind, as I imagine it, he could only think, "No. It's impossible. It shouldn't be happening. Why? I don't understand it, etc."

Horror is not the only reaction to an incomprehensible event. Another reaction is awe. An event or situation that the mind cannot take in (comprehend) will be viewed with horror or awe depending on whether it has a negative or positive aspect for the viewer. Seeing one's planes fly overhead to bomb an enemy town can be awesome. For the inhabitants of that town, however, the destruction would be horrible.

The Effect of Horror on the Personality

Let us return now to the patient I described earlier. Living constantly with a hysterical mother and a violent father was a nightmare. This was especially true because my patient felt that his parents cared for each other. Like all nightmares, all one can do is forget it. One doesn't really forget a nightmare, one passes it off as belonging to another world. One dissociates from it. This is what my patient did. He dissociated himself from his past and from all the feelings and emotions that were part of it. He cut himself off from any feeling of longing to be close to either parent, from feelings of sadness, anger and fear. This cut off was so effective that it was almost impossible to evoke these feelings. I might add that they finally emerged when his father lay dying from cancer. Faced with this tragedy, the family came to their senses.

Faced with horror, there is a tendency to disbelieve one's senses. If this tendency becomes structured in the personality, a split is engendered between what one thinks and what one senses or feels. The person doesn't trust his senses. He acts solely on the basis of the logic of his mind. He behaves as if he has feelings, which he does on a deep body level, but there is no immediate connection between the behavior and feeling.

The wails he uttered were like those of Jews at the wailing wall, an expression of the horrors he had experienced. But where the wailing Jews sensed the horrors their people had lived through, my patient was cut off from that sensing.

Persons who have gone through such experiences have an unreal quality in their personality. One senses this quality in them when they talk about a past that makes the listener shudder but which is recited in a calm, unemotional voice. The only major distortion of the body is often a discrepancy between the expression of the head and that of the rest of the body. Head and body do not fit together. There is another important feature in these people that is not easy to spot. Their eyes do not make contact with you. They do not have the empty or far-away look of a schizoid or schizophrenic individual. They are cut off from feeling, rather than withdrawn. I shall discuss this aspect of the problem again.

It is important at this point to inquire how common is this problem. What sort of horrors have patients experienced as children.

Let me say that it is much more common than we would tend to think. Here are some examples.

Another young man whose feelings could not be reached related that his mother was a Christian Scientist. In due time she became a leader in this movement. When he was young, she was a devout believer. As such she responded to all the child's feelings, distresses and illnesses with the attitude that one had only to believe in Christ and everything would be all right. But there was a hardness and insensitivity in her. She not only alienated the boy from his father but gave him no warmth. The horror of the situation for the child lay in this lack of sensitivity and warmth, in the almost complete absence of human feeling in the mother. In the child's eyes she was inhuman and, therefore, monstrous. Living under her control, domination and will must have been a nightmare for this patient.

I heard a similar story from another man who was himself a psychologist. His father had left when he was three. His mother became a religious fanatic and completely ignored the child. There were older brothers but this child felt himself to be a stranger. He was afraid of his mother and passed many years in lonely desperation. Here, again, the horror was in the absence of warmth and human feeling towards a child who needed and expected this kind of response. When I saw this man, he had a beatific expression on his face but no feelings. In both of these cases there was the marked discrepancy between the head and the body.

Recently I heard a girl describe her background as one of horror. Her father was an ambitious executive with one of the large corporations and completely immersed in his work.At home he was cold and detached. Her mother had had a nervous breakdown when this girl was young. She had been hospitalized. When she came home, she was treated as an invalid and the child had to take care of her. The mother had a number of psychotic episodes which the patient witnessed. Once again the horror resided in the absence of human contact among the members of the family. It surprised me that this girl recognized the quality of her situation but, then, she had a schizoid personality not an *as if* personality. She had not cut off the horror as a means of surviving.

In another case the mother of this patient was an alcoholic whom her father treated with undisguised contempt and hostility. At the same time he made no serious effort to stop her drinking. Sex was somehow involved in this situation, too. I suspect that the mother's drinking was the occasion for sexual relations. This became the pattern of my patient's behavior who identified with her mother. But the patient was not aware of the horror in a home where self-respect and respect for the other person were conspicuously absent.

I have heard many other tales of horror from my patients. One young woman told how she watched her grandmother put a pistol to her own head and threaten to blow her head off if her husband didn't stop drinking. Any serious threat of suicide by a parent is always a horrible experience for a child. Perhaps even more horrible is the experience of living with a dying person. Death is a horror for all young children.

Such specific instances of horror are less harmful to the personality than a situation of persistent horror characterized by a lack of human warmth and feeling in relationships where such good feelings are natural and normal. The inhuman quality in such relationships is beyond a child's comprehension. This quality creates an atmosphere of unreality. In such an atmosphere the child functions as if in a dream from which he hopes to awaken some day. When he or she grows up and gets out of the situation, the mind treats the whole experience as a dream—as if it didn't really happen.

It is hard to become excited about something that "didn't really happen," which explains why it is equally hard to evoke any emotional response from these patients in the therapy. But the effects of this kind of experience are more insidious.

When reality becomes tinged with an air of unreality, the mind protects itself against the confusion by distrusting the senses and the feelings. It denies their validity and operates only on the basis of logic and rationality. True, the logic and rationality presuppose the existence of feeling, but behavior does not stem directly from feeling. The person acts as if he had feelings but the feelings themselves are not evident in the actions. There is an inhuman or unreal quality about such people and they, in turn, become "monsters" to those who need and have a right to expect an emotional response from them. The inhumanity which has a horror to them as children produces an inhumanity in them which becomes a horror to the next generation.

The Treatment of this Problem

Generally, the presenting complaint of persons who have gone through the kind of experiences described above is depression. They become depressed when the illusion that they can stay above the horror of their own lives collapses. Unfortunately they are not aware of the illusion or of the horror in their lives. This makes treatment quite difficult. We have also seen that any attempt to reach their feelings is strongly resisted.

On the other hand, they have an awareness that something is amiss and they are depressed. They need our help and are asking for it. But how can we reach them. If the therapeutic approach is psychological, they use logic and rationality to block an appreciation of their problem. If the approach is physical, i.e., body work, they go through the motions as if they had feelings and then deny any feeling or meaning to the body experience. However, since no other approaches are available, the therapist must use both of these approaches to the best of his ability, bearing in mind the defenses he will encounter.

No therapy really depends on the approach to the problem. The important agent in every therapy is the therapist, the understanding he brings to bear on the problem and his sensitivity and warmth as a human being. These factors are crucial in the treatment of this problem. The unreality in the patient is confronted with the reality of human feeling in the therapist and this confrontation can set in motion the forces for health in the patient.

It seems to me that the therapist must respond to the patient's predicament with two sets of emotions. One is sympathy for the patient's dilemma coupled with a sincere desire to help. The second is anger at the patient for his denial of feeling and his lack of human warmth. The anger cannot be put on, it has to arise spontaneously. It should not be used as a therapeutic device; it must represent a genuine response to the monstrosity of unfeeling behavior in a situation that is loaded with the potential for emotion. In this case anger is the true expression of the therapist as a *real* human being, i.,e., one who has a feeling for life.

The specific physical block in this type of personality is in the eyes. We have an expression that says "Seeing is believing." The opposite is equally true. If one does not see it, one need not believe it. Seeing can be avoided by not letting the eyes take in expression and meaning. The eyes are used mechanically as camera lenses. They allow the picture to register but strip it of any emotional significance. This was done early in the child's life to protect it from seeing the horror in its situation. Once instituted, however, the block becomes generalized. If a person cannot see horror, then he can neither see beauty, nor sadness, anger, fear or love. And, of course, he can't allow these feelings to show in his own eyes.

It is imperative, therefore, for the therapist to establish eye contact with the patient. This is not the place to describe the various procedures and techniques for doing this. The important thing is to know that in opening up the patient's sight outward, one opens up his sight inward. In this personality it is, perhaps, the most important way for the patient to gain insight. I might add that to open up a patient's sight outward, I have him look at my eyes and try to take in their expression.

The block in the eyes is related to the dissociation of the head from the trunk. Tensions at the base of the skull and in the back of the head serve both to dissociate the head and to block the energy flow to the eyes. Considerable work has to be done on these tensions to restore the energetic flow from the body into the eyes and the perceptual centers of the forebrain. At the same time, consistent work has to be done on all other aspects of the therapy both analytically and physically.

The Cultural Horror

The horror that is found in homes is a reflection of a similar horror in society at large. To understand this statement we must bear in mind that horror is directly proportional to the lack of human feeling in relationships. This aspect of horror is more important than the violence which is rampant in our cities. It is more important because it affects everyone and gives rise to violence. The latter at least is real for the perpetrator of the violence. It may be his only way of breaking the spell of unreality that overhangs a city like New York.

I was born and grew up in New York so the city was home to me. But in those days it did not have the impersonal character it has today. I lived in a neighborhood where people knew each other personally. Through our little dealings we were intimate with the small shopkeepers who served us. A conductor collected nickels on every street car. One could say "Good morning" to him. An iceman delivered ice each day. We didn't have many comforts but we had many human contacts. And we had time. I recall a snowstorm that stopped all business activity in the city for four days. Nobody complained. We enjoyed the snow. Today if that should happen for one day, it would be a calamity. The business machine has to be kept moving and human feeling doesn't count.

Walking through the same city now, I don't recognize it. The aluminum and glass skyscrapers have an unreal quality for me. The litter and the dirt give one the sense that the city is decaying, as it really is. The rush, the hustle, the traffic have a nightmarish quality. People feel isolated. They live in cubicles, rarely speaking to each other. No one trusts another. Every person lives in a private world as people do who are committed to a mental institution.

But it is not only the impersonal aspect that is horrifying; it is the loss of human values. The only value that counts in New York is money. How much money do you make and how much do you spend? It is not the poverty that is dehumanizing; it is the filth and the indifference. It is the destruction of personal dignity. It is the vulgarity, the pornography and the filth. No one cares because caring is futile.

Is it any wonder that the horror that is outside penetrates the home? We have no way of keeping it out. Radio and television intrude their ugliness into our sanctums. And we do not see the horror of it, for if we did, we would go right out of our minds. But we are stunned and that shows in the expressionless faces, the lack of song and laughter, the moving about like robots as if we had no feelings.

It isn't much better outside of the city, as those who live in the suburbs know: Traffic that never stops, stores that remain open 24 hours a day, and the endless gadgets that promise to improve life but force us to live in terms of unimportant details. I don't think that there is anyone who owns a car who would deny that driving is a nightmare on the highway and in the town.

And yet we must act as if this is real, as if all this was the meaning of life. Oh, yes, it's real, just as any horror is real, but it is a reality that is incongruent with human nature. If we accept this reality, we must deny the reality of the body and its feelings. This is what my patients had done and they were in trouble. If we deny the reality of this kind of life, our sanity becomes questionable. We are caught in a trap, and that, too, is a kind of horror for the human spirit.

If this weren't enough, there is the horror of drugs. For whatever reason people use drugs, and some use them to escape the horror of their lives, drugs create a horror worse than they are trying to escape from. The drug user becomes an inhuman being. He loses the feelings that we identify as human. He looks unreal. I am sure that he doesn't sense the horror of his condition, for the drugs blind him to it, but he adds to the horror around us.

Actually the horror starts the moment we are born in a modern hospital. If you have seen a modern delivery room, you can realize how closely it resembles the mad scientist's horror chamber as we have seen them in the movies. There isn't a window in the delivery room for fear that if it were left open the newborn infant might become contaminated by a breath of fresh air. The delivery table, the lights and the instruments could be used in a torture chamber. As a doctor, I have put my share of time in a delivery room and so I know what I'm talking about.

The effect of horror is to dehumanize a person when he has been exposed to it for a long time. And once he has lost his humanity he can no longer see the horror. He learns to live in it as if it were real and meaningful. He can't do this with feeling but only with his intellect. And so he learns to live in his head. He doesn't withdraw like a schizophrenic who lives in a world of fantasy. He becomes a computer dealing in numbers as if numbers were the real essences while blood, flesh and feelings were meaningless objects to be manipulated in the game of monopoly we all play.

The mind has a fascination for horror because it represents the incomprehensible. As such it mocks the logic and order in our thinking. It challenges the hubris of the human mind which must explain and reduce all forces to human proportions. As we eliminate the mysteries there is nothing left to be in awe of. We do the same with horror. We apply a law of cause and effect which robs horror of its impact on our senses and so in the end we fail to see any horror.

I have often wondered why children are fascinated by horror movies. I suppose adults are too. I have thought that it represented their need to overcome the sense of horror enough to be able to function in a world that contained much horror. And this I believe is true. But the introduction of horror via movies does not help us cope with horror. It blinds us to horror by making us assume that it is a natural part of life. We learn to accept the horror, not reject it. And we become victims of horror.

LECTURE 2: SELF-EXPRESSION VS. SURVIVAL

Introduction

While the title of this lecture is self-expression versus survival, its theme is death. This theme is implicit in the title. The concept of survival implies a struggle against death or, at least, against the fear of death. If one's energies are heavily committed to the struggle for survival, one's self-expression must necessarily suffer. In this lecture I shall explore the irrational fear of death in the personality. To explain what I mean by an "irrational fear of death," I shall give an example. Some time ago one of my patients remarked, "I just had a crazy thought. I thought that if I breathe I will die." I believe we can all agree that such a thought is irrational, one doesn't die from breathing. But we cannot dismiss it. We want to know where it came from and how it affects a person's functioning.

This lecture complements my lecture of last year the subject of which was horror. Death and horror, or terror and horror (death can be terrifying) have come to assume an important place in bioenergetic analysis as we strive to comprehend the complex dynamics that underlie personality problems.

Death is not a new theme in analytic thinking. Those of you who are knowledgeable about psychoanalysis are aware that Freud introduced a concept called the *death instinct* in 1920 in an essay entitled "Beyond the Pleasure Principle." The pleasure principle had been the foundation stone of psychoanalysis. It stated that every organism strives for pleasure and to avoid pain. Freud called it the primary principle of psychic functioning. There is a secondary principle named the reality principle which modified but did not contradict the primary one. According to the reality principle an organism will postpone or sacrifice a pleasure or tolerate and accept pain for the sake of a greater pleasure in the future or to avoid a greater pain in the future. It seemed to Freud for a time that these two principles could explain all human behavior.

In his essay "Beyond the Pleasure Principle," Freud changed his mind. He postulated the existence of a compulsion to repeat unpleasurable experiences which is "more primitive, more elementary, more instinctual than the pleasure principle which it sets aside." The main evidence to support this proposition was the insurmountable resistance of patients to giving up neurotic behavior which repeated experience had shown to be unpleasurable and unsatisfactory. He pointed out that people who were not in analysis were often afflicted by a compulsion to repeat painful experiences. Some seemed to suffer from a malignant fate which made every effort follow an old pattern. These people did not have the benefit of analysis but when psychoanalytic treatment proved helpless, Freud could only reflect on the "mysterious masochistic trends of the ego."

These reflections led Freud to the conclusion that the ultimate aim of life was death. He derives this conclusion from a view of instincts as conservative, acquired historically and tending towards the "restoration of an earlier state of things." Since "what was inanimate existed before what is living," the "goal of all life is death."

But if the goal of the journey of life is death, life is also under a compulsion not to short-circuit the journey, that is, to live life fully. Freud hypothesized the existence of two instincts, a death instinct which is related to the "ego instincts" and a life instinct which is equated with Eros or the sexual instincts. It is Eros, of course, that keeps life moving on its journey but, according to Freud, it is constantly struggling against an instinctual tendency in the organism to give up the journey and to return to the stability and peace of the inorganic condition.

It is beyond the scope of this lecture to examine Freud's thinking critically. There is much in his essay that merits deep consideration and like all of Freud's work it is brilliantly conceived. My basic objections are two-fold. One, the world instinct, itself connotes a life force. As an adjective it means "infused with some animating principle." It is, therefore, a contradiction of terms to combine it with the word *death*. Second, the repetition compulsion cannot be used to explain therapeutic failure since it is the purpose of analysis or therapy to free an individual from its grip. This means that we must continually study our therapeutic failures with fresh eyes.

This is what Reich did. His analysis of the masochistic character constitutes one of the great contributions to psychoanalytic theory. Reich showed clinically that masochistic behavior was not a primary tendency in the ego, that it did not represent a wish to suffer but stemmed instead from a fear of pleasure. This demonstration clearly rejected Freud's death instinct theory and was an important factor that led to the break between Freud and Reich. Throughout his life Reich rejected the death instinct theory. It is significant, however, that towards the end of his life Reich came up with a positive and negative life force—OR for life positive orgone energy and DOR for deadly orgone energy. He remarked on the parallel between these two forms of energy and Freud's views.

We in bioenergetics have consistently followed Reich in rejecting the death instinct theory and the idea that there are "mysterious masochistic trends in the ego." Such trends were there but there was no mystery about them. They were the result of muscular tensions that limited an individual's self-expression. In my youthful enthusiasm I was sure that working with the body character-analytically, I could resolve every case of repetition compulsion. Of course, this didn't happen. Many of my patients did not get well although most made some significant improvements. However, I did not blame these failures on a "compulsion to repeat" that was innately structured in the personality. My effort and that of most of my coworkers in our institute was and is directed to increasing our understanding of the energy dynamics in personality and to improving our skills as therapists. In following this direction I came face to face with death.

The Look and Expression of Death

I first saw the face of death in a patient many years ago. In 1948 while I was a student at the University of Geneva I did some work with a young Swiss psychologist who was very much interested in Reich's ideas. One of the maneuvers I used which I took over from Reich was the evocation of fear by having a patient open his eyes and his mouth wide. This simulates the expression of fear and in many persons it serves to bring up a feeling of fear. But with many people it doesn't work. The person attempts to smile as if to say "There is nothing to be afraid of." The attempted smile masks any feeling of fear. To prevent the smile I press with two thumbs alongside the nose while the person looks into my eyes. When I did this with my Swiss patient, I saw something that shocked me. It was the hollow face of a skull. I had removed the person's mask and was looking at the face of death. I shall never forget that face.

At that time I didn't know what to do about this expression. My treatment of this patient made very little headway. I met him a number of years later. He had become an alcoholic and was deteriorating badly.

Over the years, however, I have seen this expression in quite a few patients. When I remove the mask by pressing with my thumbs, the person's face takes on a cadaverous expression. Death stares at me although rarely as sharply as in my first case.

Another aspect of the face of death is a darkness in and around the eyes. In some persons it is always present. In others it appears momentarily as if a black curtain descended over the eyes. Homer called it "the purple shade of death." When I do see this look, I have the impression that a "sense of death" lurks in the background of the personality. In some persons the look of death is an ashen-grey pallor of the complexion. Of course, this look of death is an impression one gets and as I have become more aware of these expressions I am able to pick them up more easily. The amazing thing is that these expressions of death are not uncommon. Other bioenergetic therapists have begun to see them in a large number of patients.

The idea of death often surfaces in dreams, either as a fear of dying or of being killed. One of my patients reported that he had recurrent dreams of being hunted as an outlaw. He would occasionally dream of being shot and actually experience the feeling of dying. Another such dream was recently told me by a patient.

> I dreamed I was sleeping and the window was open about six inches at the bottom. I had the feeling that someone was at the window. I woke up in the dream and saw a detached arm reach in through the window to pet my dog to keep it quiet. I was very frightened. Then the upper half of the window opened and a big, dark figure of a man flew in over my bed. I knew that he was going to rape me and attack me and I died. Then I awoke in a state of absolute terror feeling paralyzed, unable to move. Finally I got up, still in terror, and locked the window.

When I looked at this patient as she told me this dream, I saw that she was white as a ghost. She was literally scared to death and, really, in my office she looked more dead than alive.

I should add, at this point, that I had been working with this patient for more than three years. During that time she had made considerable progress as a person and in her life. In some important ways she was a different woman than the person who first started therapy. She was more alive, more open, and more able to relate to other people. At the beginning of therapy she was aloof, detached and cool. She was diagnosed as having a schizoid problem.

In view of this history two important questions arise which need our close attention. One, was she just as scared to death at the beginning of her therapy? And, if the answer is—yes, how did she hide it from herself? Two. Why did the fear of death emerge at this time?

I believe we can agree that the basic conflict underlying the schizoid character structure revolves around the right to be. Our work and that of R.D. Laing shows that there is in the schizoid individual a fear of annihilation if he asserts his right to be. This fear actually amounts to a paralyzing terror which immobilizes him. The other side of the terror is a murderous rage or fury which he dare not express. Thus the conflict becomes—to be killed or to kill. For the schizoid individual the latter means the destruction of his mother and his own death. Thus there seems no way out of the conflict except through death.

Survival in this situation can only occur on a non-being level. In a sense, the schizoid individual survives by not really existing. He detaches himself from life, he withdraws into his head and he dissociates himself from any deep feeling. The cutting off of feeling permits survival. Since the cutting off of feeling is equivalent to the suspension of life, schizoid survival is conditioned on not living. In the state of not living, there is no fear of death since one is already emotionally dead.

This analysis gives us an answer to the second question. Death or the fear of death arises when life returns emotionally, when the person now has something to lose. We shall see that this formulation is true for other character problems.

The connection between death and sex, the rape and the attack, reflects the transference of the conflict to the father. Sometime between the ages of three and seven, very roughly speaking, a schizoid girl child will attempt to secure the *right to be* through a positive relationship with the father. This attempt will occur on a sexual level since the original reaching out on an oral level was rejected. A schizoid boy will attempt to establish a sexual relationship with the mother. These attempts invariably fail but the result is that sex becomes linked with death in the deep unconscious of the individual.

We have stated as a general principle that every neurotic pattern is a survival mechanism. Every deep analysis has shown that the child had no choice, there were, as we say no viable alternatives. It is inconceivable to me to think that any living organism would surrender any natural right, freedom or self-expression, except in the interest of survival. If we take the statement literally, that every neurotic pattern is a survival mechanism, do we not imply that every characterological problem is maintained because of a fear of death?

The realization that this was true only came to me gradually in the course of the year as I worked with my patients. In case after case, though not in every one, I heard patients say, "If I let go, I will die." I shall illustrate with two cases.

The first is a man in his middle thirties whose presenting complaint was that he couldn't speak easily. He couldn't project his voice without straining. This symptom frightened him because he was in a profession where he needed his voice. He felt that the problem was due to severe throat tensions which, he recognized, were literally choking his voice off. His body was extremely tight and his legs were so stiff that he could hardly bend them.

Early in his therapy while doing one of the falling exercises, he remarked. "What I felt when I fell was that to let go was to die." Then he related this story. "When I was 13, I was told that I had a heart condition. For a year I was afraid every night that I was going to die. I felt very sick. I had a severe pain just below my heart. I got over the illness by making a supreme effort to survive. I had to use all my will power. Later some doctor told me that the pain was due to nerves." Then he remarked, "From the waist up my body feels like a solid piece of marble."

Since 13 is a critical age for most young people, I asked him what happened around this time. He said, "I started masturbating at 12. I must have had a lot of guilt because of my religious background. There was a lot of emphasis against self-indulgence—hell fire and damnation. I was entering high school then. My older brother had been a star athlete but everyone hated him. All this hostility was turned against me.

> The doctor I first saw gave me some drugs and everything went to pieces. He said that if I didn't take care of myself, I would be a cripple, that I wouldn't live to be 21. I couldn't take a full breath. If I breathed deeply, I felt my chest would break and I

would die. I had to hold my breath. At the same time I fought the bias against me among the boys. I wouldn't let anyone know I was in pain. I held it in and covered it up. I was very religious. I associated myself in my mind with David. I prayed every night to get well and promised to be good. In grade school I was a leader among the kids. The illness destroyed me. When I was doing the falling exercise, I couldn't say the word, "die." I couldn't let it out."

In this case, in contrast with the preceding one, the fear of death was close to consciousness. The whole personality had a different structure. This patient was not detached, aloof and cool; rather he was actively engaged in a struggle against death. During puberty it was a conscious struggle in which as he says, he used all his will power to survive. Today the struggle, though less conscious, is still going on and the patient is continuing to use his will power to survive. This effort takes so much energy that self-expression is necessarily limited. On the other side of the coin, self-expression, especially in the realm of sex, poses a threat to survival.

The character structure of this patient can be labeled psychopathic because the ego through the will dominates the life of the individual. Again, in contrast, the first patient was called schizoid because the defensive position was one of dissociation and withdrawal. In this connection let me say that we use the designation psychopathic not in the sense of anti-social behavior but to denote that the psychic apparatus is used to control the body and deny feelings, which is a pathological use of this system. In the schizoid state the psychic apparatus is split off from the body and its feelings.

The question that remains to be answered is whether a fear of death underlies the other character disorders. To answer that question, I shall discuss the case of a rigid character in whom neither a schizoid nor a psychopathic tendency was much in evidence. For the purpose of this discussion I shall focus on the main area of tension in this patient's body, which was the chest. This patient's chest was over-inflated and held rigidly against the release of the expiration and the giving in to the tender feelings of the heart.

Several years of intensive work had clarified many of this patient's problems and had resulted in major changes in her personality. Despite this, the rigidity of the chest had not yielded appreciably. At this point I used a technique which I had just developed. It was a simple procedure but it could be very powerful. While the person is over the stool, I ask him to breathe out as fully as possible without forcing and to hold the air out as long as possible. The instructions are simple, "Wait until you cannot wait any longer. Try to stay with the panic that develops. The body will assert its need for air against your will." If the person waits long enough, the body will suck in the air with an audible gasp. During the next minute the breathing is free and full as the "holding" has been overthrown.

The patient went through the experience of panic and her chest wall softened as her breathing became deeper. I then asked her to extend her lips and to reach out with both hands. As she did so she began to cry and clutched her chest in the region of her heart. "The pain in my heart is intolerable," she said. "I feel that it will break." It became immediately evident to both of us that the rigidity of her chest was a defense against this pain and also against her fear that her heart would break and that she would die if the pain continued. My patient knew that she wouldn't die but against so strong a feeling the conscious mind is powerless. Where did such a deep fear come from?

Every child is born with an open heart, with the desire to love and the need to be loved. For a young infant there is no distinction between the two—loving and being loved means the closest physical contact and intimacy with the mother. If, after such contact and intimacy has been established, there is a break in the relationship, the child feels betrayed. This betrayal is felt in the heart because the child is prevented from expressing its love. The heart of the child is full of feelings that it cannot express and the pain mounts to an intolerable level. The child cries and screams but to no avail and in the end the child must lock the pain into the heart and close off in order to survive. If more children do not die of broken hearts when they experience this betrayal, it is because the rejection is not total. There is some hope.

When the child becomes older, it makes another strong move to establish a love relationship with the other parent. It will open its heart to love once more. Too often, unfortunately, there is another betrayal, that is, an initial acceptance and a subsequent rejection. Again there is the pain in the heart as if a knife were thrust in. And again there is the fear of heartbreak and of death. If the father's rejection is not total, the child will survive but to do so it has to find some way to deaden the pain. This is accomplished by armoring the chest as in the rigid character structure.

It seems that in the ball game of life three strikes are out. Having struck out on two tries for love, very few persons are prepared to risk the third strike out. They can fall in love but the move is hedged with many precautions and their hearts do not stay open for long. The defense can only be abandoned momentarily and, in view of their history, I respect their precaution.

Implications and Conclusions

Let me say here that I have not fully explored all the implications, theoretical or therapeutic, of this concept. That will take time and experience. Some ideas, however, present themselves clearly.

1. The strong resistance to change that many patients show has a logical explanation. If character change involves a question of survival and means on some deep level, a confrontation with death, it is understandable why such a change is strongly resisted unconsciously. We should not say that a patient does not want to get well. No organism wants to remain in a state of illness or dis-ease. We must recognize that not all patients are prepared to take the risk that is involved in such a change. If we are aware of this fear when we work with them, it will make for a more positive therapeutic relationship. And if we can help a

patient become conscious of his fear of death when it exists, we may be able to help them see that this fear stems from the past and is not relevant to the present.

2. Freud's concept of the repetition compulsion and the death instinct can be explained in terms of psychopathology. Why do people keep repeating the same self-destructive behavior? Why is it so difficult to learn from experience? To answer these questions, I would compare the character both psychologically and physically to a shell. To step out of character is like being born or, more accurately, reborn. For a conscious individual this is a very frightening and seemingly dangerous move to make. The cracking of the shell is equivalent to a confrontation with death. Living in the shell seems to guarantee survival, even if it represents a severe limitation on one's life. To stay in the shell and suffer seems safer than to risk death for freedom and joy. This is not a consciously thought out position. It is an attitude that stems from a lesson that was once bitterly learned and is not to be forgotten.

The lesson was an early experience in which the person actually felt that his or her life was in danger. For the person had been born and, like all young creatures, was out in the world, open, exposed and vulnerable. Survival for the mammalian infant is not automatic like the young of lower orders. It needs the care and protection of a mother or parents. When this care and protection is withdrawn, even temporarily, it represents a threat to life. How callous some parents are to the very fine sensibility of infants! Some do die for no apparent reason. We call it crib death. Others get sick ,which is a real threat to a child's life.

The retreat into the shell is a withdrawal from the world and must be regarded, therefore, as a form of dying. Survival in the shell is insured by the exercise of the will. All the child's free energy is mobilized to form this shell which will allow a limited access to life and the world and yet protect it against possible future rejections or similar trauma. The shell is the character structure, it is developed by and out of the ego.

It is the person's way of saying "It is the only way I can be in the world without risking death."

And, yet, mit is a prison. It is a form of protective custody. The ego hides and confines the helpless infant to protect it from the cruel world. This helpless infant is also the heart. This is very clear from our therapeutic work. If we reach the heart of a person, we bring to light the infant in him. By the same token, if we reach and make contact with the infant in him, we touch his heart. When he exposes the infant, he opens his heart.

There is another side to this story. The shell which can be conceived of as a womb (return to the womb—retreat into the shell) eventually becomes a tomb. The situation is truly tragic. To break out of the shell is to risk death but to stay in the shell, which is a living death, threatens one also with actual death, more inevitable but slower. One of my patients who was operated on for a carcinoma of the heart described her situation as follows: "I have always had the thought that if I succeed I will die and if I fail, I will also die." She felt deep within herself that death was her only way out.

It is conceivable that in such a situation the individual will develop a wish for death which is a resignation and surrender to the belief that death is the only way out. Some such feeling underlies all suicides. Ivan Bunin, the Russian writer, described this situation very clearly in his beautiful story, "The Elaghin Affair." But this is not the same thing as a death instinct.

3. It is logical that the issue of survival should have the highest priority in an individual's life, for all other functions depend on it. But this logic is contradicted by the behavior of many people. Not everyone chooses survival at any cost. Our history contains very many examples of people and individuals who will put their life on the line for freedom, a religious belief or their right of self-expression. Patrick Henry's famous statement, "Give me liberty or give me death." shows that survival

wasn't the most important issue for him. We regard such an attitude as heroic, which it is. But we would make a mistake if we ascribed it to a few special individuals. If human beings had not been willing to fight for their freedom with their lives, if necessary, all of us would be slaves today. True, this feeling is stronger in some persons than in others. Those who have it most strongly become true heroes.

The opposite of the hero is the coward. I would define a coward as a person who puts his individual survival above all other considerations. It is not a question of fear, for everyone is afraid when there is some threat to life. Nor would I call a person a coward if his fear is so great that it immobilizes him. Many people are so terrified that they cannot move. The cowardly act is to justify or rationalize the fear, to deny one's fear and then in face of danger to betray a trust that one had encouraged. This question is important because it is relevant to the issue of death. A hero may die a glorious death but the coward always dies an ignominious death.

When a person sacrifices his right to self-expression for the sake of survival, his very survival is endangered, not from without but from within. With the surrender of the right to self-expression the meaning of life is lost. This is not a psychological phenomenon only. Self-expression is the direct and immediate manifestation of the life force in an individual. Self-expression is equivalent to life-expression and a life that isn't expressed, isn't being lived. That leads to a slow death.

Self-expression includes all the ways an individual organism makes its presence known in the world. It is a body function, for we are in the world because we have a living body. Fantasies and thoughts are not, therefore, adequate forms of self-expression until they become embodied in some bodily action, an utterance, a movement or even a look. And the more spontaneous these actions are, the more self-expressive. Thus it is in our singing, our dancing, our touching that we most express ourselves and find our greatest pleasure and joy.

4. There are some broad philosophic questions that arise in relation to the fear of death. I shall briefly touch on one which is our tendency to make survival the over-riding goal of all our activities. This emphasis upon survival makes self-expression a luxury few can afford. The present educational system is geared in large measure to preparing young people to survive in this somewhat insane world. Self-expression as I have defined it alone is relatively neglected and often discouraged. One cannot really teach self-expression since it is basically a free and spontaneous activity. But, then, one can't teach people how to live. All one can teach is how to survive. And yet it is questionable whether this teaching actually furthers their survival. In most cases it seems to end up as a deadening process.

We carry this issue of survival to absurd lengths at the great expense to society. I have in mind the medical practice of not letting people die even though all possibility of pleasurable living and self-expression is gone. By taking away from people their right to die we deprive them of their last opportunity to express themselves. In the interest of a meaningless survival we do not allow people to die with dignity and, in doing so, we rob life itself of dignity.

In my opinion this over-emphasis upon survival has distorted much biological thriving. We tend to see the evolutionary progress purely in terms of survival. It can also be seen in terms of the increasing range of self-expression which evolutionary changes have produced. The broader and stronger our self-expression, the greater is one's likelihood of survival. Not only is one's adaptability furthered but one's ability to fight is strengthened. This theme, namely, the interrelationship between self-expression and survival is discussed by A. E. Portmann in *New Paths in Biology*. He argues that every form of self-expression favors survival and this serves a dual purpose. It is unnecessary to add that survival should favor self-expression.

5. There is an important therapeutic consideration that should be discussed. The will is a survival mechanism. By its very nature it supercedes the spontaneous and involuntary responses. It comes into operation to suspend these responses in the interest of survival. Thus the will is antithetical to self-expression. Normally the will is only used in emergency situations and for short periods of time. I used the word *normally* to denote a natural state. Whenever the will is operative, therefore, one is in an emergency situation and fighting for survival whether one knows it or not and whether it is realistic or not.

When we speak of letting go in therapy, what we mean is letting go of ego controls of the will. Unless one does this, one cannot become fully self-expressive. But letting go of the will is giving up the struggle for survival. In the unconscious this raises a risk that one may not survive. If one is afraid to die, therefore, one cannot live. And if one cannot live, one is afraid of dying. The individual is caught in a vicious cycle from which there is no escape except death.

It was written in the Bible "Only as you lose your life shall you find it." The meaning is clear. Only those who are not afraid to confront death have the courage to confront life.

9

Aggression and Violence in the Individual

LECTURE I: THE BIOENERGETIC DYNAMICS OF AGGRESSION AND VIOLENCE

The Distinction between Aggression, Violence and Cruelty

Any discussion of aggression and violence in man is hampered by the confusion which surrounds the word *aggression*. In psychiatry the word has a different connotation than it does in common parlance. Ordinarily, aggression refers to an unprovoked or hostile attack upon another person. The individual who makes the initial assault is said to be aggressive and our current morality blames him for violating the peace. One can use any amount of violence in self-defense without being called aggressive. Thus *aggression* describes an attitude of moving forward or pressing forward while *defensive* denotes the attitude of holding one's position or one's ground against an assault.

From the point of view of personality, aggression is contrasted with passivity. We speak of a man as being aggressive when he moves out or reaches out for the satisfaction of his needs. The passive individual, on the other hand, waits for something to be given to him. In a broader sense, aggression is related to self-assertion. For example, a man who reaches out in love to a woman is making an aggressive move. The passive man waits for the woman to come to him. One can be aggressive in searching for work, promoting an idea, or even meeting people.

This psychological use of the term *aggression* derives from its etymology. The root, *gress*, denotes a movement; the prefix, *ag*, describes the direction. *Aggress*, as defined in *Webster's International Dictionary*, is to move forward or towards. The purpose of the movement is irrelevant. It may be done with an affectionate or hostile intent. This meaning becomes clear if we compare it with regression or digression. To regress is to move backward, to digress is to move away from. Ingress and egress are other words which have the same stem, denoting movement. The prefix merely tells the direction of the movement.

Actually, the two meanings of aggression are not too far apart. The popular meaning limits the term to hostile movements or actions; the psychological meaning ignores the motivation. How the word came to have a sinister implication I do not know. One may hypothecate that any social system which tries to maintain the status quo will place a negative judgment upon actions which aim to change the system. Those in power will defend their position against any aggressor from within or without who attempts to overthrow their power.

Where neither power nor the ownership of property play significant roles in the relationship of individuals, aggression is a natural function. Take a small child into a toy store and observe its behavior. It will reach out and appropriate whatever toy strikes its fancy. It may even try to take a toy it wants away from another child. A child is naturally aggressive. It has no hesitation in expressing its needs and desires or seeking their fulfillment.

No animal in the wild state would survive without aggression. Very little is given to it. A newborn pup that didn't move to reach its mother's teat would die of starvation. The bitch does not insert the teat into the pup's mouth. She simply lies down beside her litter and her pups do the rest—in an aggressive manner, pushing and elbowing each other out of the way to get the best teat. Breast-fed babies are similarly aggressive.

They seek the teat with rooting movements and reach out their mouths to take it in. Bottle fed babies often are more passive. They have to wait until the bottle is given to them and the nipple is put into their mouths.

Individuals become passive because their aggressive behavior patterns are blocked by fear and training. In most homes children are forced to curb their aggressive impulses. It is "don't touch," "don't run," "wait till you're asked," etc. A child must be taught that it cannot take what it wants. This is especially true in a society organized along the lines of private property. But it is no less true in communist countries. Do you think a mother would permit her child to appropriate a toy in a Moscow department store without paying for it? Only in true communities where property is held in common can a child freely express its natural aggression.

It is in the best interests of a child to allow its aggression free rein whenever possible. It will use its aggression in furtherance of its pleasure striving and not with intent to injure another person. It will have more pleasure and, as a result, become a more independent and creative adult. If, however, its aggression is blocked, it will become violent. It will fight to restore its freedom of action. Since violence is even more forbidden than aggression, the child is left with no alternative but to become passive and submissive.

Violence: Normal and Pathological

A person's natural aggressive impulses can be suppressed but they cannot be eliminated. Life, itself, is aggressive in that it is a forward moving, ongoing process that seeks to overcome all obstacles. A sprouting seed pushes its way very aggressively upward through the earth to reach the light. As long as the metabolic activities of life continue, energy is produced to power the aggressive impulses. When these impulses are blocked from expression, the normal flow of energy is dammed, creating an explosive situation.

You have seen, I am sure, how a child who is restrained against its will struggles to be free. It will fight, kick, and scream to be free to do what it wants. Why not? It was born free; it tries to live in freedom. The same thing happens when you try to take a toy away from a child that it wants. To the degree that it is vital, you will have a violent child on your hands. This doesn't mean that parents shouldn't interfere with a child's activities. Sometimes they have to. It does mean that a child's violence is generally a natural reaction to a situation of frustration.

Violent behavior is a natural reaction when one's freedom is threatened. This is true for adults as well as children. It may not always gain one's freedom. Violence tends to be met with violence and in the ensuing struggle, it will generally be the person with the stronger force who will win. It may, therefore, be better to restrain one's violence but this decision should be based on the circumstances of a situation rather than on ethical principles. A man may surrender rather than fight if it would save his life, but he has a right to fight if his freedom is jeopardized. What one surrenders is the right to fight.

Violence can also be a pathological expression. It is pathological, that is neurotic or psychotic, when it is unrelated to the actual restraint of one's freedom. If, for example, the restraint occurred in the past, then it would be pathological to act out the violence which it provoked in the present. Similarly, if the restraint is imposed by one's parents, it is pathological to release the violence upon a young sibling. Problems arise because few parents permit a child to respond violently to frustration. The violence must, therefore, find a substitute object or be held until some later time.

Most children are forced to suppress the anger and the violence they feel towards their parents in the interest of survival. They have learned that any attempt to fight results in a greater loss of freedom. The suppressed violence remains as an unexploded bomb in the personality which must be kept under tight control. The control is achieved by muscular tensions. (A contracted muscle is not free to move) But while the violence is held in check, the individual's aggression is equally blocked, thus giving him continued cause for anger and violence and a continuing need to stay in control. This creates a vicious circle which cannot be broken except by the therapeutic procedures. In effect, the person is hung-up.

Acting out suppressed violence, that is, releasing it inappropriately, has no value in releasing a person from his hang-up. Consider the case of a father who beat his child because he defies or does not obey his commands. The father's violence has no direct connection with the child's behavior. Neither the child's defiance nor his disobedience restricts the father's personal freedom. His violence indicates that his freedom was restricted probably by his own father who demanded obedience and tolerated no defiance. In hitting his child he is "acting out" the violence that belongs to a different time and situation. The only effect of such actions is to curtail the child's freedom while the parent, despite a momentary sense of release, becomes more hung-up though quiet.

Most instances of violence that occur in family situations are due to the "acting out" of suppressed violent impulses that stemmed from childhood conflicts. I am inclined to think that the violence that erupts in social situations has a similar origin. To what extent is student violence or racial violence a manifestation of neurotic behavior? And how can one tell if the violence is a reaction to an actual restraint of freedom or is an "acting out" of suppressed feelings?

These are not questions that can be answered abstractly. Every person who acts violently believes that he has good reasons for his action. Since these reasons are emotionally motivated, it is difficult to counter them. Some help can be obtained from an analysis of the personality as it is reflected in the body structure. If a person's body shows that he is hung-up, it can be expected that his personality will contain a measure of latent violence.

The Hang-ups

A hang-up develops when a person's contact with the ground is broken or significantly decreased. Personality hang-ups occur in childhood and are due to restraints placed upon a child's natural aggressivity. To understand how the restriction of aggression leads to a hang-up, one must remember that aggression is directed towards the satisfaction of needs and pleasure. An organism derives pleasure from reaching out and taking in the source of its energy, namely, food, oxygen and sensory stimulation. It also gets pleasure by discharging its energy through movement elimination, and sexual activity. Broadly speaking, the activities of taking-in are located in the upper half of the body, the activities that involve discharge in the lower half. One can appreciate the pleasure of taking-in by watching a child suck a teat, a pacifier, or a lollipop. Its pleasure in running is no less evident.

Since aggression is a function of movement it involves the muscles of the body. Outside of the limbs the main muscle mass of the body is located along the backbone. The flow of energy or feelings upward along the back and into the head and arms leads to aggressive activities in the upper half of the body; looking, sucking, biting, reaching, vocalizing, etc. When the energy or feeling flows downward into the pelvis and legs, it leads to aggressive actions with the lower part of the body. If the flow is blocked, there is a pile-up of energy between the shoulder blades. The person gets his back up, so to say, prepared to fight for his freedom of action. This area is the center for anger, as one can observe by watching a dog's hair rise along its spine when it is angry. If this anger becomes chronically blocked, it forms the basis for the hang-up. Since the energy cannot flow freely upward or downward the person is suspended—not fully in contact with the ground below nor in full contact with the environment about him. He is literally unable to move freely.

I will describe four basic types of hang-ups that can be observed in the bodies of most people. The first is the coat-hanger type of hang-up. The person's body looks as if it were suspended from a coat hanger. The shoulders are raised in an expression of fear. He is afraid to lose control for he could erupt in an outburst of violence.

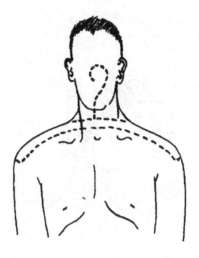

Fig. 1

The raised shoulders pull the body upward and off the ground, energetically speaking. Thus the person's freedom of movement is curtailed. This is a common type of hang-up in men who are afraid to strike out.

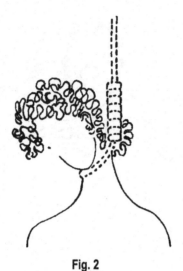

Fig. 2

    The second type of hang-up is the noose. In this hang-up the person is suspended by his neck as if there were a noose about it. People were literally hung for crimes of violence. Now they are psychologically hung-up by their fear of violence. In a body which shows this type of hang-up, the head hangs as if it were cut off from the body, which has a limp, uncharged quality. In analysis, many of these people feel that they have been strangled. Their actions are dominated by their heads and controlled by reason or logic. Their emotional life has been choked off.

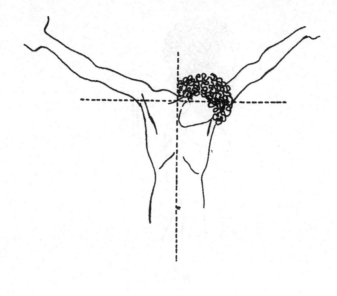

Fig. 3

A third hang-up is the cross, also seen in a scarecrow. To be hung-up on a cross is to be crucified. Jesus was crucified because he proclaimed that love was greater than authority. And even today we can be crucified for defying authority or the social rules and regulations which authority imposes. The crucified person carries a cross on his back which is composed of two systems of muscular tensions.

One runs downward along the backbone making it into a rigid vertical bar. The other extends from one shoulder blade to the other as another rigid bar. When the tensions exist in a person's body, he is immobilized as effectively as if he were nailed to a cross. His guilt is the suppression of his own violence.

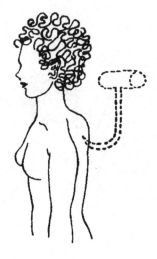

Fig. 4

I call the fourth hang-up the meat hook. The person's body looks as if it were suspended from a meat hook such as one sees in butcher shops. What gives one this impression is the knob that sticks out from the upper back just below the neck. The knob is a hard mass of flesh overlying an area of severe muscle tension. It is not infrequently seen in older women where it is called the "widow's hump." The hump represents a tremendous pile-up of anger due to the suppression of sexual feelings that goes back into childhood. The hump indicates that the body has lost its soul and has become transformed into flesh. It is also seen in men but to a lesser degree.

In all hang-ups there is a latent violence that has to be released if the person is to come down from his hang-up. This release can take place in the controlled setting of a therapeutic situation or it can be "acted out" in family or social situations using some provocation as an excuse. From what I have said earlier it should be clear that outside of the therapeutic situation no effective release is possible. It is not enough to talk about one's anger, what is needed is a physical release of the muscular tensions that create and maintain the hang-up. Bioenergetic therapy provides a proper setting where a patient can release his violent impulses without injuring himself or others. In the succeeding lectures we will describe some of the procedures used to effectuate this release.

The big therapeutic problem is that people do not feel their repressed rage and violence until they are provoked. When provoked, they direct their rage against the source of the provocation little realizing that the provocation is only the spark that sets off the dynamite. It is necessary, therefore, for a patient to feel his hang-up before the anger can be mobilized against those responsible for it. As the patient gains increasing contact with his body, the early conflicts that produced the hang-up become conscious. Their elements can be analyzed and the knots resolved.

The analysis of the repressed conflicts and the release of the suppressed violence restore the natural aggressivity of a person. We will assume that he is now grounded in his body and in the earth. His aggression will aim at pleasure; the pleasure of good bodily functioning, sexual pleasure, and pleasure to work. If, however, anyone contests his right to pleasure or prevents him from pursuing his goal of happiness, we can expect that his aggression will become hostile and that he will use all the violence necessary to preserve his freedom.

LECTURE II: THE AGGRESSIVE FUNCTIONS IN THE LOWER HALF OF THE BODY

Leg Movements

Aggression is directly connected with the function of the legs in an adult since our legs move us towards the things we want. If the motility of a person's legs is decreased, his aggressivity is reduced. He may compensate for this loss by a hyperaggressivity in the upper half of his body. Unable to move effectively, he may use his voice (yelling or screaming) to get what he wants. This is regressive behavior to the level of an infant. It may fool certain people who are unable to distinguish between pseudo aggression, which is compensatory, and true aggression. The difference is that natural aggression flows smoothly and easily while pseudo aggressive actions are hard and forced.

When a person suffers an organic paralysis of his legs, he is forced to compensate their immobility by using crutches to move about. He uses his shoulders and arms for the support and locomotion that are normally provided by the legs. Holding himself up by his shoulders he is, in effect, hung up by his shoulders, which is quite evident in his body posture. Our work does not deal with organic paralysis but with functional paralysis of the legs. The principle, however, is the same for both.

A functional paralysis of the legs is often revealed in a dream. The person dreams that he is being pursued and threatened and finds that he is unable to move his legs to escape. At this point in the dream he generally awakens. Such dreams are quite common. And such functional paralysis can occur in life. I would interpret such dreams as a recall of childhood experiences. Many mothers going to hit a child will also threaten it. "If you run away, I will only beat you harder." This threat need not be expressed in words to immobilize a child. Although he wants to flee, he is afraid to flee and so remains rooted to the spot, unable to escape his doom. If his terror is great, he may feel his legs turn to water. When such a child grows up, he will be unable to trust his legs and he will compensate their weakness by over-developing his shoulders.

A different aspect of this problem is seen in persons with thin, tight legs which remind one of bird legs. The person is continually poised for flight and all his movements are marked by flightiness. Characterologically, such persons are always running away or escaping. This unconscious attitude probably stems from a feeling of threat or insecurity in the mother-child relationship and the desire to fly upward towards the father. Whatever the cause, the effect is a loss of natural aggressivity.

There is another connection between the function of aggression and the feeling of being grounded through one's legs. This is in addition to the role of the legs to move the person. In the animal kingdom aggression among members of the same species is linked with the concept of territory. Many animals will attack in defense of their territory. The intensity of the aggressive drive is proportional to the depth of the invasion. It is weak at the periphery but becomes very strong near the center or closer to home. It is debatable whether human beings are territorial animals. Beyond debate, however, is the fact that one cannot be aggressive unless one has some ground to stand on.

Having some ground to stand on has both a psychological and a literal meaning. Psychologically, it means that a person has a good reason or cause for this aggressive action. Without the inner conviction, right or wrong, that one's aggression is justified, it would be difficult to move forward effectively. For example, a person who feels unlovable finds it very hard to reach out in affection. In another sense, the term "having some ground to stand on" means that a person feels he has the right to be on this earth and to share in the life of the earth. He feels that he has the right to be (to want, to move towards, and to take). To evaluate how strongly a person feels this right we can measure how strongly he can hold his ground. Broadly speaking, we can say that the more grounded a person is in his legs, the more strongly he can hold his ground. He will feel that he has some ground to stand on and, therefore, some standing as a person.

When a person has been deprived of his standing and of his right to be aggressive he has good reason to protest. He has, in other words, plenty to kick about. We use many modes of kicking in bioenergetic therapy to help a patient gain more feeling in his legs. Lying on a bed he will kick with his legs outstretched. This kicking is done both rhythmically and violently. It is generally recommended that patients kick 100 times a day at home to loosen up their legs. In the therapy they are encouraged to kick as violently as they can. These kicks are often accompanied by yelling such phrases as "No," "I won't," "Leave me alone," etc. Another form of kicking is to drum the legs into the bed with bent knees. One of the most effective ways to kick is arched over a stool (the kind we use for our breathing exercises.) With his buttocks on the stool and his head on the bed, the person kicks his heels alternately as if to drive someone away.

I have had patients stamp their feet on the floor as hard as they could. Putting your foot down is one way of asserting yourself. There are many other bioenergetic exercises which help a patient gain more feeling in his legs and a better contact with the ground. None of them replace the need to kick.

Ground and earth are symbolically related to the mother figure. In the earliest years our mother supports and sustains us, fulfilling the functions that the earth does for all her children. The more support and sustenance a child receives from its mother (holding, care, and affection), the more secure it feels in relation to the mother and, later, to the ground or earth. The validity of this observation can be demonstrated in every patient. It is confirmed by the study of all cultures. In less civilized societies where infants are held and nursed, the feeling of security in relation to the ground is very strong. So-called natives generally have broad, flat, and strong feet. These people also have a sense of soul, of belonging to life, of being rooted in their land.

The three areas in the mother-child relationship that are disturbed in our child-rearing practices are:

1. Holding (body contact between mother and child)
2. Bowel and bladder training
3. Erotic gratification

I have discussed the first briefly. Let us now look at the second.

Bowel Movements

Too early training to excremental cleanliness forces a child to develop control by tensing the musculature of the pelvic floor. Generally the nerve to the anal sphincter is not functional until about two and a half years of age. A younger child must, therefore, use other muscles to gain control of his anal discharge. The muscles involved are the levator ani, which forms the floor of the pelvis; the iliopsoas; and the deep gluteal muscles. Once these muscles become contracted the child develops the fear that, if he let go, his bottom would fall out. While this originally meant making a mess it later assumes the significance of a catastrophe.

There is, in addition, the phenomenon of anal spite which arises when bowel training is forced. Putting a young child on the potty with the admonition, "Stay there until you make something," evokes a natural resistance in the child which takes the form of an "I won't." Not infrequently he will soil his pants as soon as he is released. Such behavior often meets with severe punishment such as a spanking which sets up a pattern of fear, anger and spite. The outcome will always be an outward submission on the part of the child which will mask the underlying negativity which is suppressed. The unconscious suppression of negativity creates a generalized spite which says "I won't move." From an original "I won't move my bowels" the spite is broadened to an "I won't move in general."

This is an oversimplified statement of what happens. Anal anxieties can arise from the mother's feelings when she still diapers her child. If her attitude is one of disgust and distance, this will be picked up by the sensitive personality of the infant and lead to later difficulties. Shit is a very much used word in our culture, which indicates to me how obsessed we are with this function. When a child is shamed over a function which should receive little attention, it will respond with the desire to return the humiliation by shitting on the person who shamed him. It is not difficult to see why anal spite and anal hostility can have significant effects upon the personality.

Spanking upon the buttocks, especially if they are bared, frightens and humiliates a child, forcing it to tighten the superficial muscles against the pain. The child pulls his feelings out of his ass so as not to feel the hurt. This involves tension not only in the gluteal muscles but also in the hamstring muscles of the leg and in the back since the downward flow is blocked and furthers the state of being hung-up.

To get feeling back into the ass requires that the negative and hostile feelings associated with the muscular tension be activated and released. This is no easy task. The area is so far removed from normal consciousness that most people are not aware of the disturbance. Let us assume that such an awareness arises through bioenergetic therapy. What techniques can be used to release the tension?

Anal violence takes the specific form of crushing by sitting on someone. We use a simple exercise to release the impulse. The patient lies on a bed with his knees bent, and then he lifts his pelvis high into the air and brings it down hard on the mattress. The spring he gets allows him to repeat the movement rhythmically as hard as he can. The feet should not be lifted off the bed and the head should be allowed to tilt backward as the pelvis is raised. Most patients enjoy doing this exercise. It is easy and produces good feelings.

No patient can release hostility by actually shitting on a therapist bed. He can, however, verbalize this feeling. With clenched fists raised above his head he pounds the bed and says, "Shit on you." He can also be asked to name the person he would like to get back at in this way. Surprisingly it is almost everybody. Other appropriate expressions are "Don't give me any shit" and "You're full of shit." When a patient really feels free to express himself, it is equivalent to the statement "I don't give a shit." This, of course, means that he doesn't care what others say or think since he has the courage to be himself.

Kicking is also important in this problem since it will stretch and release the tight hamstring muscles. To be effective such kicking should be done with a straight leg raised to a vertical position. Above all it is important for a patient to maintain a feeling of contact with his pelvic floor. Many patients become aware of how they hold the anus tight, afraid to let it relax. Letting it out may evoke anxiety about passing wind but one soon finds that this doesn't happen. Letting the anus out as one sees it in cats and dogs opens the deep pelvis to pleasurable sensations if one is free from anxiety about this attitude.

Sexual Movements

Erotic gratification occurs first at the mouth in a nursing infant. This pleasure and gratification gradually spreads through the body and becomes focused on the genital area, some time after three years of age. In all persons a current of feeling normally flows from mouth to genital. Any disturbance of this feeling at the oral end will produce a similar disturbance at the genital end. It is not difficult to see why in a culture such as ours, where there is so little breast feeding or oral gratification, sexual difficulties are so common.

But our culture also has a negative attitude towards sexual gratification. Normal sexual curiosity and sexual play are discouraged in young children. Infant masturbation is frowned upon and the innocent exhibitionism of children meets disapproval. As a result of many forces the natural pelvic movements, which are such a delight to watch in primitive people, are inhibited in our people. Their walk is tight-assed and stiff-legged.

Normal sexual aggression or sexual intercourse produces smooth, rhythmic movements. There is no desire to pierce or to hurt in such movements. The pelvis swings loosely and freely, powered by impulses which ascend from the feet. In a person who is grounded, the impulse to movement arises from the ground. When, however, the natural flow of feeling is disturbed, the sexual movements have to be made by pushing the ass forward. These hard, compulsive sexual movements have a sadistic quality. They are hostile and what they say is "I'll fuck you" instead of "I love you."

Some degree of sexual hostility and violence exists in most people. This is the direct consequence of the loss of one's natural sexual aggression. It is also the cause of the loss of full sexual pleasure.

While it is true that this sexual hostility must be released, it is equally true that acting it out in a love relationship or on another person does not accomplish this objective. One of the techniques we use in bioenergetic therapy does help achieve this result. The patient arches over a stool and holds the back of a chair which is behind him. The stool we use is described in my books and in the chapter "Breathing, Movement, and Feeling." With his back resting on the stool at the level of his shoulder blades and his feet flat on the floor he swings his pelvis upward and downward rhythmically. He may find it difficult to do at first since his movements are restricted by strong tensions about the pelvic girdle.

As long as these pelvic swings are consciously made, their meaning is hostile. It is "Fuck you." The patient may sense this attitude spontaneously. In time, however, he will begin to identify with it. Continued work with this movement and the others described above will gradually loosen the tensions in the lower part of his body. When this happens, and when his breathing becomes full and deep, the pelvic movements take on an involuntary character. The pelvis moves spontaneously in rhythm with the breathing, moving backward with inspiration and forward with expiration. Reich described this involuntary pelvic movement as the *orgasm reflex*. It is the basis of full orgastic response in the sexual act.

I do not want to end these lectures with the impression that a few simple exercises will resolve the deep anxieties and conflicts which plague most people. Many of them do get resolved for most patients. The physical work is not only helpful, but, I believe, indispensable. Above all, it is important to know that our positive feelings are blocked by suppressed negative feelings, our affection by suppressed hostility, and our tenderness by suppressed violence. Some way must be found to help people release these feelings without "acting them out" on others. Letting them out on a bed, kicking, hitting, etc. within the context of therapy or alone can do a lot to release us from our hang-ups.

10

Psychopathic Behavior
and the Psychopathic Personality

Personality

The underlying dynamics, both psychological and physical, of the psychopathic personality have been a challenge to my understanding for a long time. In *The Physical Dynamics of Character Structure*, published in 1958, I made reference to this character and stated that I would examine it at length some day. It has taken me all these years to arrive at some understanding of this problem. In my new book, *Bioenergetics*, the psychopathic personality is recognized as one of the main character types and its basic energy dynamics and etiology are outlined. But that is not enough. There is a great need to understand psychopathia in depth and to bring our available knowledge of it to the fore. We are confronted with an increasing number of people who have psychopathic personalities or manifest psychopathic behavior and they pose an unusual difficulty for the therapist.

Unfortunately, the term *psychopathic* carries a note of opprobrium which makes it difficult to look at the problem candidly. It has long been associated in the public mind with behavior that is anti-social and this aspect has come to dominate the clinical picture. Thus, the American Psychiatric Association has dropped the designation *psychopath* in favor of *sociopath* to describe a person who acts out irrationally against society. But this leaves many aspects of psychopathic behavior outside of the concept of emotional illness. Such behavior, as we shall see in a moment, is an obvious disturbance of mental functioning, which is what the word *psychopathic* denotes. I shall, therefore, retain the term *psychopathic* for such behavior and use *sociopathic* only to describe behavior that is overtly anti-social.

What is psychopathic behavior? There are some well-known aspects of such behavior as, for example, when a person lies continually, showing no regard for the difference between truth and falsehood. We may call him a psychopathic liar, meaning that he believes his own lie and cannot tell the difference between a truth and a lie. For him, the truth and the lie are the same, which, in effect, means that everything is a lie. There is no truth and so he is not conscious of telling a lie. Another way of saying this is that the psychopathic liar believes what he says without questioning it.

Another aspect of psychopathic behavior is the almost complete indifference to the feelings or sensibilities of another person. He can do or say things that will hurt another and yet be unaware of the effect of his actions. The hostility isn't deliberate and probably because of that the psychopathic person doesn't see any hostility in his actions. He could, with reason, deny the intent, but he goes further and denies the obvious meaning.

We are also familiar with the idea that a psychopathic person has no conscience. He draws no distinctions between right and wrong or good and bad. Obviously, then, he has no guilt feelings. Thus, in extreme cases, the psychopath can steal or defraud with the attitude that it is the most natural thing to do. Of course, he knows that stealing is wrong but he doesn't see his own behavior in that light.

Because of these characteristics in his personality, psychopaths are notoriously good con people. They can make you believe that what they say is true, perhaps because they believe it themselves or because they don't believe anything. They can convince you of their innocence even when you have personally witnessed their wrong-doing. And they can win you over by their unbelievable openness.

So you are fooled. One day you realize that you have been taken and then you recognize the other as a fraud, a thief or a psychopath. You are furious, as much with yourself as with the other, because you never thought you could be such a fool.

How common is such behavior? In its extreme form it is common enough. Last year we witnessed the spectacle of a president who lied in public through his teeth, as we say, and in such a convincing manner that very many people believed him. There is no question that Nixon showed all the characteristics described above. But he was not alone. Many of his associates behaved exactly as he did.

When we analyze the dynamics that make such behavior possible, we find that they are fairly widespread in our culture. Not everyone is a psychopath, but tendencies to behave in this way exist in very many people. Lying goes on all the time with so little regard for the truth that one wonders if people are conscious of lying. Indifference and insensitivity to ethics is typical of many people in our society. Troubled by conscience? Ha! Ha! The motto is that if you can get away with it, that's all that counts. And putting on a show to influence people is the accepted strategy for succeeding.

Behavior

To understand psychopathic behavior, one must look at its extreme manifestations, simply because the problem is more clearly presented there. Let us go back to the question of lying. Doesn't it seem strange that a person can believe his own lie even when it is obviously untrue? I have heard such people relate a cock and bull story that had not a shred of evidence to support it. Weren't they aware of this? Where were their senses? The answer could be that they lost them. But from my experience of these people this isn't the case. A person who loses his senses is schizophrenic—not psychopathic. We can only conclude that the psychopathic individual doesn't believe his senses or what his senses tell him.

The only explanation that makes "sense" is that the psychopathic individual implicitly trusts his ideas but denies the validity of his senses. Let's put it this way. What goes on in his head is reality, what happens outside of his head is unreal. This is just the contrary of the way normal people function. We test our ideas against external reality, not the other way around.

If ideas are accorded the validity of reality, then there is no such thing as a lie because there is no objective truth. One has no way of knowing what is a lie and what is truth.

We say that he is unscrupulous and without conscience. But these terms have no meaning in his way of acting. If your conscience pricks you, it denotes that some deeper voice from within you is calling you to account. In the psychopath there is no deeper voice. It has been denied and negated; now it is still. He has no scruples because there is nothing within him to challenge the voice of his mind. Nothing pricks him, nothing conflicts with his ideas; no feelings upset him, no sentiments disturb him.

If he is indifferent or insensitive to you, it is because you really don't exist. He is aware of you as an image in his mind and his reactions are to the image, not to any sentient, embodied person. He can destroy you with impunity because all he is doing is wiping out an image in his mind. A psychopath is inhuman as we conceive of humanness and for that reason he is a pretty frightening character.

Of course, he doesn't exist for himself, either, except as an image in his own mind. This image is very important to him, for all his living energy is focused upon it and all his efforts are directed to enhancing it. He is fully identified with his image and when the image collapses, as happened with Nixon, all that is left is the wreck of a person.

There are a number of images in the psychopathic repertoire. The most typical is the image of power. He has to see himself as powerful and if he is not delusional, he will strive with all his being, and with whatever means are available to amass power. Not infrequently he will succeed in this, as both Nixon and Hitler showed us. Or his image may be one of youth or beauty or sexuality. Whatever the image, the drive in the psychopath's life will be to give it all the semblance of reality.

The whole thing sounds rather crazy and, in my opinion, there is a streak of insanity in the psychopathic personality. But of this, more later. Here we are trying to understand the dynamics of his behavior. The reality that the psychopath denies doesn't disappear because of his denial. He may live completely in his head, but he does have a body.

What about his body? Tell me the image to which he is attached and I will describe his body for you. If it is an image of power, he will have a powerful-looking body. If it's an image of youth, he will have a youthful-looking body. Or if it is an image of sex, his body will look like the epitome of sexuality. He is not unaware of his body; he knows it is there but it has validity only as an instrument of his mind or a manifestation of his image.

There are, also, secret images which are not directly manifested in the body's expressive form. Not every individual who is fixated on an image of power has a powerful-looking body. It may be just the opposite. The figure of Napoleon comes readily to mind. He was also called "The Little Corporal" because he was so small and yet at one time he was the most powerful man in Europe. I remember a young man only 5 feet 2 inches tall who drove the biggest car in Europe at a time when gasoline was rationed. And he was only a student. In his mind he had to see himself as big. Where most of us would say "six of one, half a dozen of another" to indicate an equality of choice, he always said "twelve of one, a dozen of another." If his physical appearance runs counter to his image, the psychopath simply denies the reality of body. It is really only the image that counts.

What is missing in the psychopathic personality are feelings. He doesn't feel the common sentiments that give meaning and direction to the lives of most people. He doesn't feel any longing or need for others and, therefore, he doesn't feel rejected or betrayed. He doesn't feel sad and, thus, cannot feel any real anger. And he won't admit that he is afraid. Since the psychopath denies that he is afraid, he will often undertake reckless or dangerous adventures, perhaps to prove to himself that he isn't afraid. It is the absence of feeling that makes the psychopath inhuman. To the degree that feelings are lacking in anyone, there is a corresponding lack of "humanness."

Yet the psychopath can put on a show of feeling that can pass for the real thing. He can become angry when his image is attacked or when he is frustrated in his attempt to project it. He may look sad when his image is rejected, but try to get him to cry and you will find that his sadness is only on the surface. The deeper emotions that come from the heart of a person like that inner voice which we recognize as conscience are sealed off from his consciousness.

He is not incapable of feeling but he is incapable of acknowledging or expressing feeling. The difference is subtle but important. In therapy one observes that his body responds with movements that one can identify as potential feeling. He looks at times as if he were going to cry or become angry, and then he will deny that he felt anything. The block must be in the connection between head and body. The head refuses to admit that the body has a life of its own. It will only recognize a body response that fits the image. The rest is denied, rejected, cut off.

What brings him to therapy?

Therapy

A 100% psychopath doesn't ever seek therapy. He doesn't trust or believe in anyone sufficiently to ask that person for help. He doesn't sense an identity with other people and this lack makes him asocial. The full-blooded psychopath is really a sociopath. He has cut himself off from any meaningful relations to others and has set himself up against people and society. Even when help is offered, he subverts the help to fit his psychopathic purposes. A good study of this personality is found in "The Mask of Sanity" by Cleckley. For Cleckley these people are really insane but their facade or mask is so convincing that insanity can't be proved.

We do not see the pure psychopaths in therapy. We see patients in whose character the psychopathic dynamic is the dominant element but not the whole picture. And we see many patients in whose character there are strong psychopathic tendencies. Since they are not pure psychopaths they are vulnerable to anxiety and depression. Their anxiety stems from the conflict between the image and feeling. They must have some feelings, otherwise there would be no anxiety. The depression is a direct consequence of the collapse of the image or illusion, but this can only happen when the image does not dominate the total personality. Another presenting complaint is a lack of feeling. Often, however, this is mentioned rather than presented as the serious problem it is. After all, the desire for feeling is itself a feeling and so in persons with no feeling at all, there is no desire for feeling.

People come to therapy with varying degrees of psychopathy in their personality. It ranges widely. Here is an example of a pretty full-blooded psychopath who consulted me many years ago. He was vice-president of a big advertising agency and he came to me on the recommendation of a business associate whom I had helped. He wanted to write a novel but he was unable to do it and he thought I could help him. The first thing he did in my office was to put his two feet up on my desk and sit back in his chair as if it was his place. I let him do it while we talked. Of course I couldn't help him. I believe I made it clear that generally if one can't write a book, it is because one has nothing to say. I think he was fascinated with me because he came for three sessions. Of course he didn't pay the bill when I sent it to him. But recognizing who he was, I sent him a letter after one week, saying that if the bill was not paid in four days, I would turn it over to my lawyer for collection. I got a check by return mail with the note, "How did you do it?"

We have said that people come to therapy not only to get well but for help in making their neurotic pattern of behavior really succeed. They want to fulfill their secret image which is an expression of the psychopathic element in their personality. But do they tell you this? Oh, no! They go along with your ideas of emotional health on the surface while inwardly they resist. If you point out their resistance, they deny it, yet the therapy doesn't move ahead. Are they lying or deceiving you? They are not conscious of lying or deceit, but then, neither is the psychopath. Only in this case there is no objective way to test the truth of their statement of intention and it is only when the secret image is exposed that the manipulation becomes clear.

Most people believe in honesty; they do not want to manipulate; they want to be straight. They are not psychopaths. But when they are under sufficient stress to make them feel trapped, the psychopathic tendency in their personality will operate. Then, they will lie to support their image without any compunction because they believe they are telling the truth. Their image is more real than the manifest expression of their body. At that time, too, they will be insensitive to you because they don't see you. The image blinds them. If the stress is less threatening, they will manipulate the situation to avoid becoming trapped. It is strange how the voice of conscience disappears when one feels threatened, rightly or wrongly.

A seemingly critical remark can bring out the psychopathic tendency. The individual will defend his behavior before he has assessed the validity of your observation. And, if he is more psychopathic, he will hold himself out as the innocent party and accuse you of hostility, jealousy, manipulation, etc.

Psychopathia and Insanity

The tendency in the psychopathic personality to deny and project, making one suspect a paranoid element in his make-up; and I personally have no doubt about its being present. This, in my opinion, is his insanity and it lies under the surface always threatening to break through the mask of sanity. It does in the case of the psychopathic murderer whose deed is insane but whose behavior after the deed is remarkably sane. It underlies the action of the forger or embezzler who has the deep conviction that he was cheated and defrauded. We shall see, later, how true that is. And it is a paranoid mechanism that motivates the anti-social actions of the sociopath.

Given some measure of underlying insanity, the psychopath must use his wits at all times to keep it under control. This means that his mind is working all the time. Asking such a person to let go of his head in order to allow some feeling to surface is equivalent to the demand that he allow himself to go crazy, become insane. In this connection we may recall that R. D. Laing believes that a person may have to let himself go crazy in order that his true self may emerge. That is pretty frightening. Fear of an underlying insanity will force any individual into a psychopathic attitude as a defense.

One will not understand this concept of the psychopathic attitude as a defense against insanity without a knowledge of the dynamic elements in a psychotic break. Two factors are important: one is an ego that is weak or insecure because it is not identified with the body or the body ego and not integrated with the feelings. The vulnerability to such an attack is set forth in *The Betrayal of the Body*. The other factor is a flood of feeling that cannot be integrated by the ego. The feeling could be fear, anger, sexuality or longing. The important thing is that the feeling is overwhelming, flooding the perceptual mind and eradicating the boundaries of the self. Any situation that weakens an insecure ego while strong feelings are evoked can produce a break.

The psychotic episode is ushered in by a state of confusion, which leads into a feeling of estrangement. Reality becomes nebulous, the person is like in a trance. In this condition the individual can express the feeling, that is, act it out. He may kill someone or himself, he may lock himself in a closet or tear his hair in grief or he can go dead to stop the feeling. In the latter case he becomes catatonic. In both cases his mind is no longer connected with his actions; he has dissociated or split off from his body and his feelings.

The psychopathic defense is to make sure that feelings never reach an intensity where they threaten to overwhelm the ego. One way to do this is to cut out every impulse so that no charge ever builds up. A second way is to deaden feeling through alcohol or drugs. And the third way is to deny any significance to relationships, thereby preventing the possibility of feeling. The psychopath uses all these means and others to prevent himself from feeling. He may abstract feeling to a cosmic level by becoming a mystic. On this level he can talk about feeling but he is talking about abstractions or ghosts, not the common everyday feelings of human beings whose life is a struggle for the simple pleasures and joy of living.

This adds up to the fact that the psychopath lacks a sense of humanity. To the degree of his psychopathy, he is inhuman. He cannot and dare not give in to the condition of being human.

What does it mean to be human? It means basically to be helpless and in need. In the most important aspects of life, a human being is helpless. He didn't ask to be born and he has no control over when he will die. He cannot choose with whom to fall in love. He is not master of his own fate. His helplessness is tolerable because all human beings are in the same boat, all share a common fate. And each one needs the others to counter the darkness, to keep out the cold, to provide a meaning to existence. We each need others to provide the light, the warmth, the excitement and the challenge of a human community. Only within the human community dare we face the terrifying unknown.

The psychopath is no exception to this human need. He, too, needs people. But he dare not— and cannot—acknowledge this need. It is too dangerous. In a moment we will consider why this is so. Here let us examine how he handles this problem.

Almost invariably one finds that the psychopath is surrounded with followers. He needs followers and he will use every trick to obtain them. He will beguile, charm, seduce, entice people to need him. He knows their fears and weaknesses since they are his own and he will promote, promise and proclaim that he will be their light, their warmth, their excitement and their challenge. He holds himself out as superior because he doesn't need anyone. And it seems that he is superior because human anxieties do not trouble him. Desperate people, frightened people and lost people will turn to him as to a savior. Hasn't he manifested that he can rise above the human struggle?

One might ask—aren't there psychopaths without followers? The answer is "No." He must have at least one follower, one devotee, one slave: she could be his woman, his prostitute, his homosexual lover. But he must have someone who needs him. He cannot be alone. The other person provides the human contact he must have, but on his terms—needing him, depending on him, worshipping him.

Of course the game would be up the moment the follower confronted his "leader" with "You need me as much if not more than I need you. You are as frightened of life and death as I am, if not more. You are so scared you dare not admit your need." I make no claim that the psychopath would come to his senses by such a confrontation. It might, however, put a dent in his ability to bewitch other helpless people who are terrified of their helplessness.

Etiology

How did the psychopath get that way? Why is he so afraid to need? What events twisted his mind?

Every individual starts life in a state of helplessness and need. An infant's very existence is dependent on others. In this respect the human infant is not different from the very young of birds and mammals. Without the protection, security, care and nurturing of the parents, these young would not survive. It is a one-way street: the parents give, the child receives or takes. That is as it should be, for a generation later these young will do the same for their offspring. And so the river of life flows downhill always.

Would you not doubt your senses if you saw water flowing up a mountain? You might say, "It's crazy, it can't be." There is a natural order to life. What can a child think if it becomes aware that the roles are reversed, that the mother is looking to the child for mothering and fulfillment. How many times have I heard patients say, "I was a mother to my mother."

Turning the natural order upside down causes an unbelievable havoc in the child's personality. The developing personality of a child goes through many stresses and strains before it becomes strong enough to cope with reality in a mature, adult way. One of the major stresses is the oedipal situation. Every child feels a sexual attraction for the parent of the opposite sex. It experiences a precocious flowering of sexuality between the ages of 3 and 6. This is in line with the development of the first or baby teeth, another expression of precocious maturity. These teeth fall out as the permanent teeth start to erupt. Similarly, the early sexual efflorescence recedes to prepare the way for the permanent sexuality of puberty.

These early experiences, sexual and others, are stressful for a child but it is biologically equipped to handle them. What it cannot handle is adult sexuality. Its sexual feelings for a parent are a natural phenomenon; a parent's sexual feelings for a child are unnatural like water flowing upstream. This, too, can happen. We can pump water up a hill but we know that it is the work of man, not nature. How can or how does a child deal with the sexual feelings of a parent directed at it? This is what we call "seductive behavior" on the part of the parent.

It can't say to a parent, "Hold on. This isn't the way it's supposed to be. Your sexual feelings are supposed to be directed towards your mate, not your child." It can't say this because: (1) the child isn't consciously aware at first of what is going on. Generally, the seduction starts quite early, often before the age of 3; (2) the child instinctively responds to the seduction with interest and excitement. It is, after all, an expression of love, albeit misplaced and destructive. And in most cases, if not all, the child had suffered some deprivation of the care and nurturing it needed earlier, and, hungry for attention and affection, it responds to the seductive invitation.

This response on the part of the child suddenly changes the situation from an imaginative experience into a real one. No longer is it an idea in the child's mind; it has become a real sexual relationship even if it is not acted out. That possibility cannot be denied by the child for whom feeling and action are closely associated. The real situation creates a real triangle. There is now the threat from the parent of the same sex who is viewed as a competitor.

The child is trapped. It cannot turn to the parent of the same sex for help, for it senses, rightly so, that it would be blamed. To give in to the seduction is insane. It is biologically incapable of integrating adult sexuality. And it cannot reject the seductive parent to whom it is now bound. The only possibility is to accept the situation and learn to play the game.

The first step is to cut off sexual feeling so that it cannot be tempted into the insanity of incest at the age of 6, for example, nor tormented by a desire that cannot possibly be fulfilled. It does this by tightening the belly and withdrawing its energy and feelings from the lower part of the body. This creates the typical psychopathic body structure with its overdeveloped upper half and relatively underdeveloped lower half. Being still subject to the seductive excitement, it must find a way to discharge this excitation. This is done through hyperkinetic activity and compulsive undertakings. Dr. John Bellis pointed out the hypermotility of the psychopathic personality.

These bodily defenses coupled in responding to the seduction are overcome by denying any sexual feeling for the parent of the opposite sex. The denial is broad, covering not only the forbidden response but also the natural, innocent and sweet feelings of the child. In denying these feelings, it also denies any need for the parent of the opposite sex. It was the need to be close to this parent that made it vulnerable in the first place.

Denial is a psychic defense but to be effective and sure it must be structured in the body. It becomes structured as a ring of tension at the base of the head that prevents any excitation from the body getting into the head. In effect, the head is cut off perceptually from the body so that the person can say, "I don't feel anything." In addition, this tension disrupts the flow of energy to the eyes so that the person can also say, "I don't see anything." Not seeing negates objective reality and leaves the individual with only his ideas and images as his reality.

Those of you familiar with my ideas about schizophrenia and the schizoid condition as elaborated in *The Betrayal of the Body* may recall that I described a somewhat similar ring of tension in that state. There are similarities and differences between the two conditions. In the psychopathic personality the ring of tension cuts off the expressive functions but leaves the motor function relatively intact.

The difference between the schizoid condition and the psychopathic condition is best explained by the distinction between terror and horror. We regard the schizoid condition as being frozen with terror. The terror is a fear of annihilation if the individual asserted his right to be. It represents an experience of rejection, generally at a very early age. The psychopath, on the other hand, is not threatened with annihilation but with castration for his sexual responsiveness. He is seduced, then blamed. He is trapped in a nightmare of horror. The situation is unbelievable; it makes no sense in terms of his original feelings of love and the desire for closeness. It has an air of unreality and like a nightmare the child tries to put it out of his mind. I would strongly recommend reading the chapter on "Horror" to understand these distinctions.

There are other factors that enter into the etiology of psychopathia. The child is subject to considerable manipulation, often amounting to brainwashing, as the parents or parent try to instill in the child's mind an image of how they want him to be. Often there is a power struggle going on in the home which the child is conscious of and in which he is used by one parent against the other. A mother will often use her son to put down her husband, for example, with the remark, "You, I hope, will not turn out to be like your father." Who is he supposed to be like—his mother? Or a father who feels himself to be the underdog at home will elicit his daughter's sympathy and thereby subtly turn her against her mother. I will, in another context, discuss the social factors that corrode and undermine the harmony and stability of family relations to prepare the terrain that breeds psychopathia and schizophrenia.

If you want to see a clear picture of the perverse relationship between a mother and son, see the movie, "Alice Doesn't Live Here Anymore." I think you will be shocked at the evident seductive behavior of the mother. The language between them is unbelievable. Strangely, most people viewing the movie find it cute, which is beyond my comprehension.

The Psychopathic Maneuver

Cutting off sexual feelings, not necessarily genital ones, withdrawing one's energy upward, especially into the head, and denying feeling, constitute the first step in the defensive process. If it should stop here, the child would find itself isolated, having lost its vital connection to its parents. Isolation leads to withdrawal, turning inward and the development of a fantasy life to replace an intolerable and unbelievable reality. The end result would be an autistic state verging on schizophrenia. Some relationship must be reestablished with a parental figure. This can be accomplished in two ways, by becoming submissive to the seductive parent but without feeling, i.e., letting one's self be used, or by becoming dominant. The true psychopath follows the latter course and it is the one I shall investigate here.

The true psychopath turns back to the seductive parent, but in a reversal of roles. He or she becomes the seducer, promising to fulfill the parent but withholding satisfaction. It is an astute maneuver. Having denied and cut off the feeling of need the child becomes objective. He can now see the need of the seductive parent which now can be turned to his own advantage. Just as he was trapped by his need, the parent can now be trapped by her need. The same applies to the relationship between a girl and her father. The child learns the rules of this game. You can promise anything because fulfillment is impossible. This is important to understand. The promise is an irresistible bait just as long as fulfillment is impossible. This deduction follows logically from the nature of the situation. When a parent is seductive with a child, that parent doesn't want any real sexual contact with the child. He or she would deny any such intent and rightly so. The taboo against incest is powerful in these persons. Should the child make an overt sexual move toward the parent, he or she would be severely rejected. Even normal physical closeness becomes suspect. What the parent wants is the excitement, unfortunately at the expense of the integrity, both moral and physical, of the child. If fulfillment were the natural outcome of the relationship, the excitement would disappear.

The child becomes a psychopath by playing this game. He promises to be the ideal child, to be his mother's darling or her father's darling, then disappoints the parent. Of course, as soon as the parent is disappointed, he promises anew, which hooks the parent even more strongly because of the earlier disappointment. Holding both the promise and threat of disappointment over the parent, he can extract from the parent everything he wants. He has the parent in his power.

As long as he has his parent in his power by this maneuver, he is protected from the double danger: isolation and withdrawal into depression and insanity, on the one hand, and surrender to the forbidden impulse leading to incest and insanity, on the other. At the same time, his need for closeness and relatedness is somewhat met albeit in a perverse way. The two individuals in this relationship are not committed to each other by a feeling for the other, but involved with each other out of their need to play the game.

The promise that the child makes is rarely expressed in words. It is contained in the image which may or may not be manifested in the form of the body. It is expressed in the manner, in the bearing of the person, in his attitude, and in his tone of voice. Part of the child's personality tries to live up to the image, part of the personality rebels. The strength of each of these two forces varies in different individuals. In some the rebellion is very strong and the person will act out his negative feelings to negate the image. In others the rebellion is subdued. The quantitative factors in each case are unique and have to be determined from a careful analysis of the person's history. And the degree of psychopathy in each personality also varies according to the inducements and pressures to which the child was subject.

There are psychopaths who rise to high positions in government and industry while others become gangsters, criminals and murderers. Some are successful but most are failures, petty crooks, con men, gamblers, pimps, adventurers, etc. We tend, of course, to focus upon the more notorious examples, because they are more interesting to study and read about, but it would be a grave mistake to regard the problem of psychopathia as limited in its obvious manifestations. People who are psychopaths or who have strong psychopathic tendencies can be found in every field of human endeavor and activity. And our own profession of psychiatry or psychotherapy is not immune to them.

How does one recognize a psychopath or psychopathic behavior? This question merits some comment. Associated with that question is another directed to his dupe, his victim, his follower. Who is ensnared by the psychopath? And why are people so vulnerable?

The Pretender and the Gullible

I have characterized the psychopath as a person who makes a promise that he is not committed to fulfill. That means he lacks integrity. That's a good term, but it requires definition. We can only understand what integrity is by examining the psychopathic personality bioenergetically.

I noted that the basic problem is not an inability to feel or to sense but a denial of the body, of feeling, and of the senses. Of course, the denial by the ego in its perceptual function creates a lack of feeling on the perceptual level, but this lack is not the same as that which occurs in the schizoid state. The denial by the ego is a pathological condition in the psychic apparatus which justifies the term *psycho-path*. In schizophrenia we are dealing with a split or dissociation. The feeling is not denied; it is, however, not connected. The schizophrenic individual also lacks integrity, but we can excuse him because he claims no virtue for this lack as the psychopath does. I shall return to that statement a little later.

The lack of integrity in the psychopathic structure is caused by the mind turning against the body, or to put it better, by thinking which negates feeling. The lack of integrity is manifested physically on the body level. The head isn't connected energetically to the rest of the body. Sometimes it doesn't fit the body. We sometimes see the head of a child on a mature body or the head of an adult on a childish-looking body. Sometimes it is a small head on a large body or vice-versa. The cause for this disturbance is the ring of tension at the base of the skull.

Another physical characteristic is the pulling upward off the ground so that the feet are not energetically connected to the ground. Often this pulling upward blows up the upper half of the body so that it is markedly out of proportion with the lower half. Whether this is the case or not, the psychopathic character isn't connected to his feet. The function of being grounded in reality and on the earth is severely disturbed.

Two other physical functions are disturbed in a typical manner. The first is genitality. It is not connected to the sexuality of the body let alone to any feeling of love. Because of this the psychopath doesn't know the difference between fucking and loving just as he doesn't know the difference between lying and telling the truth. He will claim that there is no difference because he truly cannot perceive one. I am not castigating a person who has sex without love any more than I would pillory a person for lying. The point I want to make is that it is psychopathic not to recognize or sense the difference.

Physically, the cut-off between genitality and sexuality is caused by a ring of tension around the root of the penis. Stanley Keleman made me describe this ring of tension. I don't remember if he related it to the psychopathic problem. Actually it is a psychological form of castration related to the oedipal situation. The same ring of tension exists in women. The child pulls its sexual feelings out of its belly, not out of the genitals, to overcome the incestuous seduction. Working physically in this area, one can palpate the tension and evoke severe anxiety. It is the Achille's heel in the psychopathic structure.

334

The second function that is disturbed in this structure is seeing. I mentioned earlier that the psychopath doesn't see you. You are only an image in his mind. His vision is intact, so he sees your image on his retina. But seeing is more than recording an image. It is a sense function, which means that he senses you. It involves recognition. In this connection it is interesting to note that some primitive people in Africa use the expression "I see you" as a form of greeting. In effect it says "I recognize you as a person."

Here, too, it is meaningful to compare the schizophrenic eye disturbance with the psychopathic one. In *The Betrayal of the Body*, I pointed out that the schizoid individual sees but he doesn't look. Looking is an active process which involves focusing the eyes to take in the image. Normally when a person looks at you, he touches you energetically with his eyes. He makes eye contact. This function is blocked in the schizoid structure. The psychopathic individual does look at you, he may even fix you with his eyes, but the contact is limited because the look is distrustful or controlling. In the paranoid personality, the distrustful look frequently has a searching quality. But much as the psychopath looks at you, he doesn't see you. His mind denies the reality of his sensing, he cannot surrender his preconceived images.

These physical characteristics of the lack of integrity in the psychopathic personality are infallible. Unfortunately it requires considerable experience to recognize them. Necessarily we must rely on an analysis of his behavior and attitude to conform our impressions.

On the psychological level the lack of integrity is reflected in a lack of moral principles. To our present culture, a term like *moral principles* may seem old-fashioned and authoritarian. In our rebellion against imposed principles we overlook the fact that there are natural principles. Truthfulness is such a principle. Young children are naturally truthful. They weren't taught it. They will learn later to tell a lie, but hopefully they will not lose their ability to recognize the difference between a truth and a lie. And, hopefully, they will hold to the principle that honesty is the best policy.

I discussed the nature of principles in the last chapter of *Bioenergetics*. I said that principles develop when feeling and thinking are integrated. This integration is missing in the psychopathic structure because any feeling that fails to support the image or that doesn't accord with the thinking is denied. One can say, therefore, that the psychopath is a person without principles. That is the essential nature of his character structure. The corollary of this proposition is that any individual whose behavior is not governed by inner moral principles is psychopathic.

In place of principles the psychopath substitutes power as his guide and goal. This is not a new concept in our thinking. We have recognized for a long time now that psychopathy is characterized by a drive for power. Often it is openly avowed; in many cases, however, it is artfully concealed behind a facade of justice, righteousness, morality, etc. Let us not forget that the psychopath is the great pretender. He knows how to play the game and put on the show. Well, then, how can one distinguish between the pretense and the real thing, between a statement of principles and principled behavior?

There are several important criteria one can use to make this distinction. A man of principle will eschew power or he may even reject it when it is offered. Power corrupts the soul and easily undermines one's principles. A psychopath, however, welcomes power in the name of his principles. How dishonest can one be? I could elaborate on this idea but it would take us too far afield of this presentation.

Another criterion is the use of any means to achieve an end. The dictum that "the end justifies the means" is a psychopathic byword. Political revolutionaries proclaim this dictum and under its aegis they often commit very inhuman actions. Many business people secretly uphold it and engage in practices that, if they are not illegal, are deceitful and dishonest. It is a pernicious doctrine. Anyone who follows it behaves psychopathically. A quick analysis will expose its psychopathic nature.

The end is always a preconceived idea. It is an image of a future condition, a goal not yet realized. I am not against goals, ends or images. To have a goal is not psychopathic. To use any means to achieve it is. It means that one must sacrifice his principles and deny his feelings. That is the psychopathic attitude.

I would equate the end with the head, for the head is the end of the body. The means would be the rest of the body. Is the body to serve the head or is the head in the service of the body? I believe you know by this time which order I would regard as psychopathic.

A third criterion in recognizing psychopathic behavior is the absence of humanity. I mentioned this earlier but it is worth expounding. Every decent person knows how difficult it is to be open, straight and honest in our culture. It is always a struggle to be faithful to one's principles in a society that has abandoned that view of man. He knows, too, that human beings are not perfect creatures. It is typical of a straight person that while he may hold high standards for himself, he is tolerant and understanding of the common human weaknesses and faults. Psychopaths are deficient in this human quality. They are not only lacking in it, they hold it in contempt. They are above the common human weaknesses, they are special. This sense of being special carries with it an arrogance that offends human sensibility. It is in my opinion the characteristic quality of the psychopath.

Now, what about those who are the dupes, the gullible, the victims. One of my patients called them the "suckers." Obviously, there are plenty of those around.

The sucker is a person who goes for the bait, the promise, and gets hooked. The word *sucker* denotes an oral element in the personality, a lack of fullness. This lack is very widespread in our culture where sucking, i.e., breast feeding, is a rare phenomenon. However, it doesn't explain the sucker's gullibility. That gullibility derives from exposure to a psychopathic parent who promises, doesn't deliver, then promises again.

"If you are a good girl, mother will love you." So you try, but it doesn't work. The love is not forthcoming. You are frustrated, become restless and irritable. There is a fight, you are blamed, you cry and the promise is made again. "If you are a good girl, mother will love you." What choice does the child have? It has to believe in the promise because it is helpless and dependent. It has to believe in the possibility of love. The child does not know that conditional love is not love at all, that a promise of love is an empty gesture. One shouldn't promise to feel because feelings are not subject to conscious control. It is the kind of promise that can't be fulfilled. It is therefore a psychopathic maneuver.

Psychopathic maneuvering on the part of a parent results eventually in a psychopathic response on the part of the child. It is impossible for a child to be what a parent wants him to be. No one can change his essential nature. No child can be totally good, for the submission to the parent's wishes evokes a rebellion against the parents. The effort to be good creates the bad. As long as a person is allowed to be who he naturally is, there is neither good nor bad, neither submission nor rebellion.

The problem of psychopathy is not how or why it developed but why it persists. What are the economic factors in the personality that maintain the gullible attitude into adulthood? Why doesn't a person come to his senses after he has left the seductive and rejecting situation of his childhood? I shall answer these questions in the next section.

The Treatment of Psychopathy

You have all heard that the psychopathic character is very difficult to treat. That should not be a surprise. Since we know that he doesn't believe in anything, it is irrational on our part to assume that he believes in therapy or has any trust in the therapist. However, if he does come to therapy, it means that he is desperate, that he needs help whether he acknowledges it or not. It also means that he has some sense that things are not right with him, some feeling of unhappiness.

The worst thing a therapist could do is to promise him that one can help. As soon as he extracts a promise, his psychopathic defense is activated. He knows that game well and can play it better than the therapist. He knows you can't deliver and so he sees you as no different from himself. In that case he questions whether you have anything to offer him and he will drop out as soon as he becomes bored with your therapeutic game. Or he may stay to learn the rules of this new game, which can make one feel superior to all the desperate souls who come to him in need. The therapeutic role can easily be used to serve the psychopathic position.

Since most people in our culture have some degree of psychopathy in their personalities, it is a wise rule of therapy not to make any promises. I make it a policy not to require that a person coming to me for help commit himself to the process. He is free to leave and I am free to terminate the therapy if either is dissatisfied with the relationship. Of course, we will discuss our doubts and distrust of each other, but I have confidence that if he senses that the therapy does not help or offer him something real, he will stay. Along this line, if one senses that the client has some clear psychopathic tendencies, it is well to express one's doubts immediately about what the therapy can do. Simply taking such a person for treatment without expressing this doubt can be construed as an implied promise to help. That's pretty tricky.

We get around this issue by focusing upon our client's problems, both physical and psychological. We can point out the disturbances on the body level and we can try to help him get in touch with them. But as for changing anyone, that we can't do. An honest statement is "It's your body and I can't do it for you." That's absolutely true. We can't breathe for him, and we can't feel for him. And we can't straighten out his twisted personality. We can only point out the twist and explain why it became that way, but we cannot make him accept our explanation.

In helping a person understand his way of being, it is important to know what we call the secondary gains from the illness. On the psychological level, these supposed gains keep a person locked into his neurotic functioning. At the end of the last section, I asked: What factor in the personality maintains the gullible attitude into adulthood? We should start with the question: What keeps a psychopath committed to his way of being, since he often recognizes, as we do too, that it is a frustrating, self-defeating and empty life style? The answer is, being special. For the gullible person, it is the desire to be special coupled generally with the secret image of being special too.

The psychopath is a person who believes he is special. The seductive situation that created the problem convinced him that he was, indeed, special. He was special to the seductive parent, he was needed and used by that parent both emotionally and sexually. And it was conveyed to him that he had the power to fulfill that parent. What a position to put a child in! It awakes and reinforces his infantile sense of omnipotence at a time in life when he should be moving toward independence, separation and reality.

I would not be stretching the truth by saying that the child in this situation is looked upon as a little god. And he may even be worshipped as one by his parents. At the same time he may be used and abused. We do this with our gods, too.

This view of the psychopath may surprise you, but look at the parallels. A god can do no wrong, he has no conscience, he doesn't believe in anything but himself. A god is above human considerations of right and wrong, truth and falsehood. He is also above the common human weaknesses and vulnerability, which is the position of the psychopath. He doesn't need others, they need him. He is omnipotent as the psychopath believes himself to be.

It would be interesting at this point to examine the history of some notorious psychopaths like Manson and Hitler. I believe one will find that on some deep level they see themselves as god-like. What we see is the devil in them. That examination, however, must be reserved for another occasion.

I have not worked with this kind of psychopathic individual. My patients may be considered ordinary law-abiding persons. Yet in almost every one I found a secret image of being special and a secret wish to be special. And I wonder—who in our culture doesn't have it. Some say it openly. They want to be treated by me as "special." They resent it if I treat them like the rest of my patients. Others do not acknowledge it, but I am sure it is there.

In the musical, "The Fantastiks," the ingenue sings a song asking to be special. That is her deepest wish. To be special—what an image.

It almost makes up for all the pain one has suffered. Unfortunately, the realization is missing that it is also the cause of one's suffering. Ah, yes! We would like to be free of the pain and the suffering, but we do not want to give up the image of being special.

Some years ago Dr. George Greenberg gave a lecture for the Institute on the family in which he said that the role of the family was to make the child feel special. I never forgot that remark. At the time I was impressed with the astuteness of his observation and I thought, "Why, yes, that is the positive side of the family role." I suppose I was still identified with my own image of being special. And that, I learned, turned out to be my own hang-up. Today I see "being special" in a different light—as the biggest obstacle to emotional health.

To work this problem out with patients, I ask them what it means to be special. Each person has a unique image. One woman said, "I always thought I was special. I was told that I could achieve anything I wanted if I tried hard enough, and I believed it. Isn't that the American way? I achieved a lot but it didn't work in the important areas of love and sex." A psychiatrist said, "For me, being special means knowing all the secrets of people's lives. I sit behind the scenes like a director or producer knowing everything that's going to happen."

For a schizophrenic patient, being special was identified with being ill. Working with her, I discovered that she was a fairly competent person but her specialness required her to deny her strength and her abilities. She kept them hidden probably for some other special person who would need her and love her. This denial had not caused her illness. She was not playing sick, she was sick. The denial prevented her from getting well.

Let's look at the other side of the picture. What does it mean not to be special, to be common, that is, like all the other people. I contrast these two attitudes for my patients and they are often quite surprised at the comparison.

What is common to all people are their bodies. Each is alike and functions alike. The "special" person must deny his identification with his body for that would make him like every one else. He must also deny his feelings, for they, too, are common. Everyone loves, hates, is angry, sad, frightened, etc. The person who is special is identified with his thinking and his images, which are unique. Common to all humanity and even to the animals is sexuality. To be special requires that one surrender one's sexuality.

Being special sets one apart, for we refer to the ordinary people as the "common" people. It is not a derogatory term except to people who see a virtue in being special. The common people have each other, they belong to the human race, they share the common struggle, they are not alone. The special person is bound or tied to the person who made him feel special. This becomes very clear in the course of the analysis. The child who was not special is free. The special person is not only apart, he is above the others. I mentioned this aspect of psychopathy earlier. The common people are grounded in the reality of life. And while the special person is fated to live out a special destiny, the common people laugh and cry, have pain and pleasure, know sorrow and joy. Simply stated, they live their lives, the special person imagines his living.

There is one quality we associate with "common" which the special person lacks and that is common sense. It is the lack of common sense that makes a person gullible, just as it is the denial of common sense that forces the psychopath to invest his life and energy in the futile attempt to fulfill an illusion.

Recall the story of Jonathan Livingston Seagull. He was a "special" bird. He was not interested in the squawking and squabbling of the other seagulls. He wanted no part of their fighting for a piece of rotten fish. He was above it. Where the other birds were content to remain within the limits of ordinary seagull life, he was obsessed with the idea of transcending those limits. So he went off on his own to become pure spirit, interested in pure love—no sex, mind you.

Which would you choose? The psychopath didn't choose to be special. He was forced to give up his sexuality and was offered in its place the image of being special. It was a poor bargain but he had no choice. Having made the deal, he is reluctant to renounce it, since one cannot give him back his sexuality. But if he doesn't give up his image of being special, he has no chance of recovering his sexuality.

I cannot leave this subject of specialness without recognizing that people do have special gifts. We are each unique with abilities and talents that are different from those of other persons. But this does not make us feel special since we recognize that being unique and having special gifts is common to all people. And we don't seek our identity in our specialness but in our commonness. Can you say "I am a man" or "I am a woman" or "I am an American." If you can, and when you do, you will be amazed to discover that one's identity derives from the common heritage.

For many people, seeing the problem clearly expressed in this way is a help. Whatever health there is in a person will fight for feeling and sexuality. Therapeutically, the problem of psychopathy has to be handled on two levels. Through the physical work with the body, the person is helped to get in touch with his feelings and his sexuality. This requires a focus on the underlying sexual anxiety, namely, the fear of castration. The psychological work helps him see the deception that was practiced on him and the illusions to which it gave rise.

Conclusion

The psychopath is known as a manipulator. All his manipulations and maneuvers are designed to make other people recognize him as special. All of us who manipulate others have this end in mind. And all of us who have a secret image of being special are manipulators.

Making promises one cannot fulfill is manipulation. The political arena is full of such people today. But the field of therapy is not without its psychopathic element. Approaches that promise to save you, to fulfill you, to actualize you, etc., are manipulations designed to make you see the promotor as special. He has the answers. He knows the way. He can tell you or show you how to do it. And people fall for these promises because they are lost and desperate. But they go for them also because in their secret hearts they see themselves as special. It doesn't matter that it didn't happen to others. (We refuse to see the failures.) It will happen to me because I'm special.

I don't know if Bioenergetics falls into this category. I hope not. I didn't promise you anything tonight. I have tried to share with you my understanding of the problems we have in common.

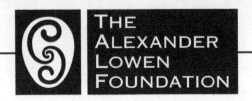

Bioenergetic Analysis for life, love, health, and environment...

The Alexander Lowen Foundation is a U.S. based international non-profit organization dedicated to archiving, preserving, and expanding the work of Alexander Lowen, M.D.

Online Therapy and Learning

International **Workshops**

Bioenergetic **Bodywork**

Publishing of Lowen books

We invite you to learn more about Bioenergetics and the works of Dr. Alexander Lowen at:

www.LowenFoundation.org

Vermont, USA
Call 802-338-2866
Email info@lowenfoundation.org